Healing
Nutrition

DATE DUE

OCT 1 0 1996	APR - 8 2002
	MAR 2 1 2003
NOV - 8 1996	APR 1 5 2003
MAR 2 9 1997	NOV 0 7 2004
APR 1 7 1997	
MAY 2 3 1997	
SEP 1 7 1997	
NOV 2 4 1997	
DEC - 8 1997	
FEB 1 4 1998	
OCT - 5 1998	
OCT 1 6 1998	
NOV 2 9 1998	
MAR - 4 1999	
MAR 1 9 1999	
APR - 3 1999	
JAN 2 6 2000	
Mar 9/00	
NOV 2 3 2000	

BRODART.   Cat. No. 23-221

Healing
Nutrition

LYNN KEEGAN, PhD, RN
Associate Professor
The University of Texas
Health Science Center at San Antonio
School of Nursing

Director, BodyMind Systems
Temple, Texas

Delmar Publishers

I(T)P™

An International Thomson Publishing Company

Albany • Bonn • Boston • Cincinnati • Detroit • London
Madrid • Melbourne • Mexico City • New York • Pacific Grove
Paris • San Francisco • Singapore • Tokyo • Toronto • Washington

NOTICE TO THE READER

Cover Design: Spiral Design
Cover Illustration: Kirsten Soderlind

Delmar Staff
Publisher: Diane L. McOscar
Senior Acquisitions Editor: Bill Burgower
Assistant Editor: Debra M. Flis
Project Editor: Judith Boyd Nelson
Production Coordinator: Barbara A. Bullock
Art and Design Coordinator: Mary E. Siener
Editorial Assistant: Chrisoula Baikos

COPYRIGHT © 1996
By Delmar Publishers
a division of International Thomson Publishing Inc.

The ITP logo is a trademark under license.

Printed in the United States of America

For more information, contact:

Delmar Publishers
3 Columbia Circle, Box 15015
Albany, New York 12212-5015

International Thomson Publishing Europe
Berkshire House 168-173
High Holborn
London, WC1V 7AA
England

Thomas Nelson Australia
102 Dodds Street
South Melbourne, 3205
Victoria, Australia

Nelson Canada
1120 Birchmont Road
Scarborough, Ontario
Canada, M1K 5G4

International Thomson Editores
Campos Eliseos 385, Piso 7
Col Polanco
11560 Mexico D F Mexico

International Thomson Publishing GmbH
Konigswinterer Strasse 418
53227 Bonn
Germany

International Thomson Publishing Asia
221 Henderson Road
#05-10 Henderson Building
Singapore 0315

International Thomson Publishing—Japan
Hirakawacho Kyowa Building, 3F
2-2-1 Hirakawacho
Chiyoda-ku, Tokyo 102
Japan

1 2 3 4 5 6 7 8 9 10 XXX 01 00 99 98 97 96 95

Library of Congress Cataloging-in-Publication Data

Keegan, Lynn.
    Healing nutrition / Lynn Keegan.
        p.   cm. — (Nurse as healer series)
    Includes index.
    ISBN 0-8273-6868-2
    1. Nutrition   2. Nursing   I. Title.   II. Series.
RT87.N87K44   1996
    613.2 — dc20
                                                        94–44097
                                                        CIP

INTRODUCTION TO NURSE AS HEALER SERIES

LYNN KEEGAN, PhD, RN, Series Editor

*Associate Professor, School of Nursing,
University of Texas Health Science Center at San Antonio
and Director of BodyMind Systems, Temple, TX*

To nurse means to care for or to nurture with compassion. Most nurses begin their formal education with this ideal. Many nurses retain this orientation after graduation, and some manage their entire careers under this guiding principle of caring. Many of us, however, tend to forget this ideal in the hectic pace of our professional and personal lives. We may become discouraged and feel a sense of burnout.

Throughout the past decade I have spoken at many conferences with thousands of nurses. Their experience of frustration and failure is quite common. These nurses feel themselves spread as pawns across a health care system too large to control or understand. In part, this may be because they have forgotten their true roles as nurse-healers.

When individuals redirect their personal vision and empower themselves, an entire pattern may begin to change. And so it is now with the nursing profession. Most of us conceptualize nursing as much more than a vocation. We are greater than our individual roles as scientists, specialists, or care deliverers. We currently search for a name to put on our new conception of the empowered nurse. The recently introduced term *nurse-healer* aptly describes the qualities of an increasing number of clinicians, educators, administrators, and nurse practitioners. Today all nurses are awakening to the realization that they have the potential for healing.

It is my feeling that most nurses, when awakened and guided to develop their own healing potential, will function both as nurses and healers. Thus, the concept of nurse as healer is born. When nurses realize they have the ability to evoke others' healing, as well as care for them, a shift of consciousness begins to occur. As individual awareness and changes in skill building occur, a collective understanding of this new concept emerges. This knowledge, along with a shift in attitudes and new kinds of behavior, allows empowered nurses to renew themselves in an expanded role. The Nurse As Healer Series is born out of the belief that nurses are ready to embrace guidance that inspires them in their journeys of empowerment. Each book in the series may stand alone or be used in complementary fashion with other books. I hope and believe that information herein will strengthen you both personally and professionally, and provide you with the help and confidence to embark upon the path of nurse-healer.

Titles in the Nurse As Healer Series:

Healing Touch: A Resource for Health Care Professionals

Healing Life's Crises: A Guide for Nurses

The Nurse's Meditative Journal

Healing Nutrition

Healing the Dying

Awareness in Healing

Creative Imagery in Nursing

DEDICATION

To my inspiring, long-time friend
Barbara Dossey, RN, MS, FAAN
a dynamic, nutritionally balanced, physically fit,
living example of body-mind-spirit integration.

C O N T E N T S

P R E F A C E

It has been said that educators teach what they want to learn and authors write what they want to know. In the case of this book, I have been blessed with the opportunity to learn much about the fascinating subject of nutrition. As I have researched this subject, I have become more aware of the calorie, fat, vitamin, and mineral content of my meals and snacks. Going to a dinner party or dining out has become an entertaining challenge of self-discipline as I learn to stay within newly recognized dietary guidelines.

As I spent the year with this topic, I began to understand why there are so many diseases related to nutrition. As I increase my knowledge about this topic, I realize how and why most Americans are practically illiterate when it comes to nutrition. There is so much valuable, lifesaving information to know, yet as a society we give so little formal attention to nutrition. I marvel at the concern given to the details of a high school education, the specifics and parameters of each individual course and the outcomes that purport to prepare us for life. Yet America's educational system does not adequately prepare us to care for our bodies.

As physical organisms, we are composed of millions of biochemicals. The daily input of replacement biochemicals in the form of nutrients is critical to the optimal functioning of our marvelous bodies. Unfortunately, much of the general public and many health care professionals have been negligent in attending to our nutritional health. With newfound attention to this subject as we round out this century, each of us will become increasingly aware of acquiring information not only to prevent disease but to maximize a vital, productive life. Each of us, armed with nutritional knowledge, can serve as a resource person to others. As a collective whole, we can meet the objective of increased health and vitality for all peoples.

My hope is that the numerous books and articles I have devoured to expand my understanding of this subject have become an amalgam of practical wisdom to assist you, the reader, in expanding your breadth and depth of useful information on the subject of healing nutrition. It is my additional desire that this material will be of value for both you and your clients.

A C K N O W L E D G M E N T S

Fortunately there are always people who are present at the right place and at the right time to aid and abet us on our path through life. While I worked on this book I had the good fortune to have a devoted editor who continually encouraged me to write. Because of our growing professional relationship, I now think of Bill Burgower as a friend as well as a senior administrative editor for Delmar Publishers, Inc. Assistant editor, Deborah Flis, provided the leadership for the invaluable editorial assistance that facilitated the development of this book; many thanks to Deb.

I wish to acknowledge my older, svelte, and healthy daughter, Catherine, for her contributions and insights, especially in the chapters on dieting and emotions. Thanks to the other members of my immediate family, Gerry and Genevieve, who always support my need for the time to work on my special projects.

Special thanks to Wanda Whitely, MS, RN, a teaching colleague who gives me enthusiastic encouragement no matter what I am writing. Two former graduate students, Peggy Weiser, MS, RN, CNM and Martha Burke, MS, RN, CNM, learned well in class and became excellent manuscript reviewers. Their remarks provided the necessary information for a smooth transition from a rough draft to the manuscript you now read. Kimberly Moore, MS, RD (registered dietitian), provided invaluable assistance in validating technical and scientific information about the specifics and details of this increasingly esoteric science—healing nutrition.

I N T R O D U C T I O N

Nutrition is our most fundamental need. We all require food and drink for basic maintenance and growth. You have probably heard the old adage, "You are what you eat." Not only are we what we eat, we are also influenced by how we eat, with whom we eat, when we eat, where we eat, and why we eat. As bio-psycho-social-spiritual beings continually interacting with our environment, we are influenced by, as well as exert an influence upon, our world.

Everything we do has meaning. Understanding the meaning of our daily habits, rituals, and behaviors comprises the nature of our conscious and unconscious philosophical striving. Seeking to understand nutrition and our attitudes about food is of utmost interest and concern in today's society. Why, where, when, and how we eat rank as some of our most primal questions. This book seeks to answer some of the questions about why nutrition is important and how best to provide ourselves with the optimal food for a healthy, healing life.

This book is *not* about nutritional therapy for hospitalized patients or for clients in severely compromised clinical conditions. It does not address total parenteral nutrition, enteral nutrition, or subjects such as nutritional support of the ventilator-dependent patient. This book does not contain material on diabetic exchange diets or ethical issues regarding withholding or withdrawing nutritional support. Rather, this is a book about healing nutrition to optimize a robust life.

The content is geared to maximize learning about the whys and wherefores of obtaining and eating high-quality, life giving foods. It is designed to offer ideas to reinvigorate both the nurse and the client. You should read this book when you are not ill, nor necessarily well, but rather in the ho-hum state of living in which so many countless millions of us spend our days. Most of us do not lack zest for living because we are nutritionally deprived, but rather because we have not optimized our potential in many realms of life, including the realm of nutrition. This book will aid you in discovering why you should pay more attention to healing nutrition, including issues such as what you are eating, where to find different food products, and the influences of why, when, where, how, and with whom you are eating.

In this book, you will find both facts and ideas. As nurses, we need to understand domains based on scientific models. Consequently, within this text, you will find tables and figures on which to build your knowledge base. On the other hand, much of our motivation and impetus for change comes from another dimension, a dimension emanating from the subconscious and/or superconscious. Based on this truism, understanding healing nutrition from the paradigm of holism is also emphasized within the text. Lastly, the theme of healing is the backbone of this work. Therefore, all the content is directed toward gleaning information for self-healing and assisting others in their healing processes.

THE IMPORTANCE OF HEALING NUTRITION

1 WHY HEALING NUTRITION?

HOLISM

We are holistic beings. As such, we live on multiple interacting planes. Nutrition plays an active role in each of our component parts. For example, one who eats wholesome, living, broad-spectrum foods is more likely to have a healthy physical body. One who has a healthy physical body is more likely to develop or possess a healthy spirit, mind, and emotions. Consider figure 1.1, which depicts a holistic template that demonstrates the interrelationship of each of our holistic component parts.

Each of our daily actions affects our total health. Because of the holistic aspect of our being, each system has a direct or indirect effect on every other system. We are not static physical forms but human beings who live in continual flow and change and are constantly renewing ourselves in all areas. As we evolve, it is not only our bodies that change. We are so connected that changing the body simultaneously affects the mind and spirit. For example, when we begin to shed unwanted pounds and tighten muscle groups, we feel simultaneous lifts in our spirits and mental outlooks. On the other hand, when we accumulate more and more weight and nothing fits, we feel accompanying drops in zest and sluggishness of our spirits. Once we become aware of these concepts we begin to realize healing in any one area of being is related to all aspects of the self.

	BODY	MIND	SPIRIT
BODY	body body	mind body	spirit body
MIND	body mind	mind mind	spirit mind
SPIRIT	body spirit	mind spirit	spirit spirit

FIGURE 1.1 Body-mind-spirit template.

Reprinted from Keegan, L., & Dossey, B. 1987. *Self-care: A program to improve your life.* Used with permission of Bodymind Systems. Temple, TX.

CASE STUDY | *Nadia's Story*

In 1976, Nadia Comaneci was the first woman in Olympic gymnastic history to make a perfect score. She won one bronze medal and three gold medals. In 1979, she came to the United States to compete in the World Gymnastics Championships. Everyone expected a brilliant performance, but after a few competitive rounds, she was hospitalized with what was called a minor infection on her hand. Due to a delayed healing response, she had to remain hospitalized. Newspaper reports from the Fort Worth Star Telegram (December 10, 1979) revealed that Nadia had been eating only one full meal every 2 days and snacking on occasional fruits and vegetables to lose a few pounds to maintain her slim, lithe figure.

It had taken tremendous teamwork to get Nadia into this world-renowned position; yet the team had neglected the need for optimum nutrition. Although the team included someone who was responsible for nutrition, the gymnastic coaches were concerned with maintaining Nadia's body weight and continuing her long practice hours. As a result of the imbalance, Nadia's body became so depleted that it was unable to fight off a simple infection. The malnourished body is susceptible to infections because the immune defense system and the antibody response are decreased. (Burtis, 1988, p. 11)

A NEW RESPECT FOR FOOD

Our growing respect for the innate powers of food is actually not new; it is simply reemerging. Pharmacopoeias of ancient Egypt, Babylonia, Greece, and China were based on food. It was Hippocrates who proclaimed, "Let your food be your medicine and let your medicine be your food." Twelfth-century Jewish physician/philosopher Maimonides recommended chicken soup as a remedy for asthma. Garlic, mustard seed, and other herbs and spices collected in herb gardens or from the countryside were used medicinally by healers for centuries.

It was not until the modern pharmaceutical industry arose in the nineteenth century that we placed the obvious behind us and became enamored with manufactured stop-gap methods. Now as health costs have skyrocketed and the harmful side effects of drugs are becoming increasingly apparent, there is a resurgence of interest in dietary moderation and treatment with natural foods and herbs. For example, many of us might take an antacid if we have discomfort from overeating. Before this pharmacological era, we would not have had the medicine to mask this sort of symptom. We would probably have been more careful the next time not to overindulge and suffer from its untoward effects. With each passing year within this decade, there seems to be increasing awareness of the benefits of moderation and the considered use of food to prevent illness as well as to heal maladies.

THE CIRCLE OF HUMAN POTENTIAL

The dance of life involves many possibilities. I like to envision people as beings of wholeness and as such I am attracted to the model of the Circle of Human Potentials (figure 1.2). This model is comprised of six areas: physical, mental, emotional, spiritual, relationships, and choices. A circle is an ancient symbol of wholeness. The circle in this model has six separate but equally important parts. When any part is incomplete, the entire circle loses its completeness because all parts create the whole.

FIGURE 1.2   The circle of human potentials.

Reprinted from Keegan, L., & Dossey, B. 1987. *Self-care: A program to improve your life.* Used with permission of Bodymind Systems, Temple, TX.

All of our human potentials constantly interact. When we treat our physical bodies with respect by feeding them properly and care for them by ingesting only healthy foods, we begin to change other aspects of our beings. As we become stronger by eating nutritiously, exercising, stretching, and making other physical improvements, we begin to become healthier and happier. This then impacts our other potentials.

We can learn through conscious effort how to enhance health and decrease the symptoms of disease. The idea of consciousness must be central in the continued development and understanding of our human potential. When we think of wholeness, we not only affect our attitudes toward others, but also affect our understanding of our connectedness of body, mind, and spirit.

SUMMARY

The importance of a good diet is not new; what is new is the affirmation that incidences of chronic diseases have dietary links and that a good diet can help prevent, as well as treat, disease. Although some of us may need to enhance our food intake with isolated nutrients due to biochemical individuality, no supplement can take the place of a basic, well-rounded diet. Hippocrates was right—food is our best medicine.

Reference

Burtis, G., Davis, J., & Martin, S. (1988). *Applied nutrition and diet therapy.* Philadelphia: W. B. Saunders Co.

2 THE MEANING OF FOOD

"Hey Mom. What's for dinner?"

"I'm starving. Honey, let's go out tonight."

"It's my birthday and I want to eat the whole carton of ice cream."

"I'm taking five pounds off and that's all there is to it! So, no, I will not join you for lunch."

OVERVIEW

For each of us, food carries meaning. The meaning may vary from year to year, season to season, or event to event, but food is always coupled with meaning. Historically, homemakers have brought families together around tables at dinnertime. In many homes, special weekly meals are still planned following Sunday or Sabbath religious services, and celebratory meals follow major life events such as baptisms, weddings, and even funerals. Any way we look at it, food is used to commemorate significant life events. However, not all of the associations are positive. Consider, for example, the last time you were angry or sick. Do you recall a lack of appetite? Remember times of sadness or depression. These events are often coupled with anorexia, or lack of appetite. However, some of us experience the opposite reaction during times of grief and eat more than is normal. Suffice it to say that food is directly associated with both positive and negative emotions and the events linked to those emotional times. The meaning of food is inexorably intertwined with our bodies, minds, and spirits.

CHOICES

The joy of healthy nutrition is that we are part of it. We get to choose what enters our bodies. But before we can hope to select a diet intelligently, we must first learn about the values of foods, what minerals and vitamins they contain, and how our bodies use minerals and vitamins to give us great health and long lives. Every time we go to the store or sit down to a meal, we make a choice as to what to eat. We learn to base these choices on what our bodies need as well as on our feelings, desires, and conditioned responses. The more information we have, the greater our ability to understand the meaning we attach to food and to make healthy choices about it.

Foods have power. Foods transfer their power to us when we digest and assimilate them. One of the basic premises behind the ability of food to heal is that food is comprised of organic chemicals just as we are. The body's chemical structure is strikingly similar to that of seawater. However, the chemical elements in our bodies are structured in a more highly evolved order.

Unlike medicines, food enables us to build up or tear down the tissues of our bodies. When we eat well, we build strong, healthy bodies, but when our diets are defective, we tear down our bodies by destroying vital tissues. There is a power within each of us that can work miracles if we provide our bodies with the minerals and vitamins they need.

It has been known for a long time that no cell lasts longer than 7 years. What few of us know is that the majority of cells do not live nearly that long. For example, we grow several fingernails in a year; dermal skin cells take only 2 years to be replaced. Furthermore, physiologic chemists say our bodies do not contain a blood cell that is more than 14 days old. Even more amazing is that we rebuild a new heart every 30 days. That means we have a new start in life every month, a new beginning in which to provide the proper nutrition that can revitalize our bodies and our lives. By eating properly we can possibly add 10, 20, 30, or even 40 years to our life spans. Each day brings a new opportunity for a fresh start.

Our organs are destined to self–repair, but they need opportunities to do so. They will mold junk food, doing the best they can with what we give them. When we properly balance our diets, however, our bodies begin to respond. When taken into the body, every bit of food does one of three things:

1. It goes into the building of new bones and tissue.

2. It supplies the energy for gland secretion and for cleansing.

3. It merely passes through the digestive and elimination organs.

The number of calories we ingest means little unless the calories come from a proper balance of food. Without a continuing variety of nutrient-enriched foods, good health cannot be achieved.

ATTITUDE

What we want to strive for, along with healthy nutrition and balanced lifestyles, are positive mental attitudes. We are all born with the potential to live long, healthy, and happy lives, but we usually fall short because of two main reasons: (1) misinformation and (2) inconsistency. Most of us simply do not adhere to lifelong regimens of wholesome diets and regular exercise. All of us need moderate regular exercise along with good diets. The point is to be consistent. It is not what we eat or drink or how we move occasionally that determines our levels of health. It is what we practice daily that determines how long and how well we will live.

We would all improve our lives tremendously if we applied what many corporations are ingraining in the minds of their employees: quality, consistency, and performance. We, as individuals, need to be conscious about the quality of our lives, know what it is that we want, have a plan for obtaining it, and have the energy to do so.

A life filled with quality work, positive thoughts, loving friends, and activity tends to strengthen our natural immunity to germs, viruses, and negative hereditary influences. A positive attitude works hand in hand with good nutrition. Healing nutrition can work, rebuilding our bodies from the inside out as we open them to the interrelationship of mental, spiritual, and emotional aspects of food's curative powers. The effectiveness of healing food has been clinically proven by research and thousands of individual case histories. The way to begin is to feel a true harmony with life in our hearts, a harmony set free by the knowledge about what will bring quality into our lives every hour of every day that we spend on this earth.

Every acute disease episode is a healing crisis. It results when the body struggles to free itself of toxins. Nature does her best to keep the body clean, but we must help. Every insect and animal has a natural instinct for self-preservation. The farther up the animal chain, the more this instinct is lost. Ironically, as animals, our instincts are often safer than our intelligence. When an animal is sick it eats nothing, or it eats only grass. In effect, it purges its body of toxins. Many foods do produce remarkable short-term benefits. However, it is only with consistent proper nutrition and exercise of the body, along with the proper state of mind, that we can achieve a state of wellness that safeguards against imbalance in our systems and contributes to disease prevention. It is certainly possible that healing foods that can prevent an illness can also cure an illness.

QUALITY OF LIFE

Ask yourself: On the whole, am I as healthy as I can be? Are those with whom I live and work healthy? Before you answer, visually remember the last time you were in a committee meeting or at a large conference. In your mind's eye, look at the people. Were they physically fit? Did they look tired and haggard? What did their skin look like? Were their eyes clear and bright? And what about the older people? Were they energetic and full of life or worn out and tired of living? Now, how about you? Are you filled with zest and vitality, or is there room for improvement? Is your quality of life what you want it to be? The easiest place to begin is with your physical body, with what you put into your mouth. Most of us want quality of life. Through a change in dietary habits, we can achieve it. The remarkable by-product is that, with effort, not only do we improve the quality of our lives, but we are also likely to increase our satisfaction with our lives.

LIFE EXTENSION

The search for the fountain of youth is as old as mankind. From ancient culture to modern civilization, extending the human life span has changed from an elusive dream to a present-day reality. The secret of maximizing life expectancy and living youthfully well into old age, the 90s and beyond, is not found in a synthesized new drug or bionic body part; the key is the foods we eat.

I was first exposed to the idea of life expansion through the theories of Durk Pearson and Sandy Shaw (1982) described in their book *Life Extension*. My initial reaction was that their method seemed risky: too many supplements and too little scientific validation. It is the basic idea of the theory that stayed with me, and I continue to explore it.

To many, old age brings senility, incontinence, and chronic illness often with concomitant pain and misery until death finally occurs. Who wants to live like that? Chronological age may not, in fact, have to be linked with cellular age. Cellular age can be defined as the age of the cells in our bodies. What if being 80 meant looking and feeling like you were a 40-year-old who has the vitality of a 20- or 30-year-old? Imagine living well past 100 without any illness or disease because your cells function as if they were decades younger. Think about having multiple careers and pursuing new hobbies or enjoying romantic interests well into your 90s and beyond. Consider what that could mean. How many people work hard all of their lives and never get to enjoy the money and leisure for which they labored? Imagine being young and vital at 65 and living a full and healthful life.

One of the goals of this book is to help you learn to live healthfully to your maximum life span. This means not just adding years to old age but stretching out the periods of youth and middle age so that at 80 calendar years, the cells in our bodies function as those of a youthful 40-year-old, full of energy and vitality. Whatever our reasons may be for wanting to live younger longer, it may actually be possible to reverse the symptoms of aging and extend our life spans by doing one very simple thing: Make the decision to consistently adjust our eating habits.

Food is the giver of life. Sickness does occur because of genetics, germs, or just plain bad luck, but the vast majority of all illness is the result of how we choose to live our lives. The results of the choices we make regarding the food we eat, most of which we have more control over than any other factor, determine how long we will live and the quality of life we will have. Until you have experienced it, you may understand this principle on an intellectual level but not necessarily on the deeper emotional level. In other words, until we feel more alive and healthier than we have ever felt, these are just words that have little meaning. The secret to living younger longer is not about transplanted organs, surgery, or synthetic drugs; it is about strengthening the physiology within our bodies. Life extension is about erasing the errors of years of eating lifeless, highly processed foods and feeding our bodies the vital nutrients they need on a cellular level to increase vital functions and ward off infection and disease.

Human Evolution

Humans evolved over millions of years, and this evolution was shaped by many factors, including climates, habitat, and the ability to adapt to the environment. Early people were hunter gatherers, living off of fruits, nuts, and plants and hunting animals for food and clothing. Their food was rich in nutrients and loaded with the necessary life-giving energy. The fact is that the human species has remained relatively unchanged for the last 40,000 years. Our physiological makeup is the same as that of our Stone Age ancestors. For the most part, Stone Age people were lean, strong, aerobically fit, and almost totally free of the chronic diseases that cause 75 percent of all deaths in the United States today. Changes in human nutrition and exercise patterns have contributed to cancer, heart disease, diabetes, hypertension, obesity, and even the tooth decay that we have today. In the Stone Age, death was seldom caused by degenerative disease because the average life span of Stone Age people was shorter than that of contemporary people. Instead, death likely came from confrontations with animals, life-threatening injuries, or natural disasters.

Forty thousand years ago, people lived in seminomadic tribes. They moved with the seasons, following game, water, and plant foods. They were lean and strong and dependent upon their stamina and strength for survival. Although their diet was occasionally insufficient in quantity, they usually had enough to eat, and most importantly their food was rich in life-giving nutrients. Those who survived the assault of accidents and infections could look forward to a long and fit life, untroubled by the degenerative diseases that afflict modern humans. The point is that our Stone Age ancestors did not die of the same diseases that recently have caused most of the deaths in the United States, and yet, physiologically, they were identical to us. The primary differences between them and us, other than some environmental factors, are the activity levels and foods we eat. Through various processes over the last 40,000 years, our food supply has changed. The way our ancestors lived was relatively the same for over a million years, but then something happened. This event was not the Ice Age or a meteor striking the planet. No, this event was far more significant because what happened biologically changed the earth and altered the destiny of humankind forever.

About 10,000 years ago, some of our ancestors abandoned their age-old hunting and gathering way of life for a more settled existence based upon agriculture and, eventually, upon animal husbandry. Humans began to grow their own food. Like a genie let out of a bottle, powerful and unprecedented forces were unleashed: forces unlike those that had controlled the ecology and evolution of plants, animals, and microorganisms during the preceding 3 billion years. This event, known as the Neolithic Revolution, transformed our planet.

Once introduced, agriculture prevailed as the leading pattern for human subsistence and was a very efficient way of feeding larger groups of people. With agriculture, humans began to flourish, and as a people, we began to control our food supply. We had more time to develop our cultures. Civilizations were created. Science, art, and the quest for enlightenment expanded. The planet was transformed. Today we are the beneficiaries of these changes.

As humans discovered agriculture and began cooking, processing, and storing food, modern health problems slowly began to surface. Diseases that never existed began to afflict human beings. We had better shelter, warmer clothing, and most importantly, plenty of food. Where were these new diseases coming from? Remember, for millions of years humans evolved by eating only what they could gather, forage, or kill. The relationship with food was based solely on survival. Think about that for a moment. Before agriculture was introduced, humans ate only to survive. Our bodies' evolution was the result of food that was present in the natural world. In this natural world, life exists based only on what it needs to survive. Now, with the sudden abundance of food, that perfect relationship that exists only in nature was changed as people began to eat for pleasure. They ate because they wanted to eat. When the desire to eat changed from need to want, the natural state of human health was never the same again.

As people became more skilled at raising crops and domesticating animals, foods became plentiful, and the variety of choices increased as well. These choices were based on a new variable: taste. Then, inevitably, came the intentional manipulation and creation of foods based upon markets for things that tasted good. Remember, for millions of years, humans ate foods that were available from hunting or foraging, foods that were rich in nutrients to which the human body had carefully adapted, foods that the body was programmed to digest with the help of nature. Selection and choice were limited and driven by hunger; the purpose of eating was to survive.

Think of this connection between taste, evolution, and the manipulation of our food supply. The taste of food is merely a biological mechanism that tells the brain what foods to eat and what foods not to eat. In general, foods that had energy and nutrients to sustain life were foods that tasted good. Nuts and berries that were too sour or too bitter were poison, or at least unripe, and were therefore not good nutrient choices. These foods were discarded because they were not pleasant to eat. By using the sense of taste, humans unconsciously selected the proper foods that would nourish them and discarded substances that would not nourish them. What is truly amazing is the power of our sense of taste.

In the natural world, survival is the first priority. Every function of every living organism has one primary overriding objective—survival. Taste is one of the survival mechanisms developed over millions of years to help us select nutrient-rich foods and to eat them in sufficient quantities to ensure survival. So, what does it all mean? What do taste buds and cavepeople have to do with living to a healthful old age? The answer is "everything." Taste drives us to pick certain foods. Evolution formed a powerful connection between our taste buds and our brains, and this happened not in the last 100 years but over millions of years. When we eat something that tastes good, our bodies signal our brains that this food is necessary for survival and our brains tell us yes, that is good, eat more, eat as much as we can, because in the natural world, our next meal may be a long way off. That was then, however, and this is now.

The difference today is that foods that taste good are not always good for us. As we humans became skilled at growing food and domesticating animals, we literally altered the natural world. Foods were genetically altered in large part to satisfy our sense of taste. We learned the art of hybridization to a degree that many of the foods we used to eat as a species no longer exist today. Grains such as corn and wheat, as well as the livestock we eat today, are not the same as those of 1,000 years ago or even 100 years ago.

The objective of the modern food manufacturing business, like any industry, is to create products that will satisfy markets and create profits. To meet these objectives, the food industry has created foods that taste good so that we will buy them. On the surface, this may seem relatively harmless. If you think about it, the result of millions of years of evolution, in which there was this perfect relationship between humans and their food supply, suddenly changed. The slightly salty taste of a natural root or nut, the semisweet flavor of a wild berry, or the warm and succulent taste of wild game all send signals to our brains, triggering a desire to eat. This perfectly natural biological mechanism that was designed to ensure survival is now being used to select foods with exaggerated flavors. What is amazing is that we are talking about three basic tastes: the tastes of fat, sugar, and salt. Think about it. A thick, juicy steak, heavy butter and cream sauces, and rich desserts all contain excessive amounts of fat, sugar, and salt, foods that did not even exist a thousand years ago. Why do humans crave these kinds of foods, and why do we become obsessed with eating them? To better understand, let us look at each taste in terms of human nutrition.

Fat   Fats are a necessary part of our diets. They contain essential fatty acids that are needed to formulate hundreds of chemicals in our bodies. They also make up the components of our entire hormone system. Fats are needed to prevent inflammation, lubricate our joints, and form the linings of our cells. Certain fats help remove cholesterol from our arteries, transport certain vitamins to hungry cells, and help our immune systems fight disease. Fat is also used as stored energy. When fat is not used at the time of consumption, it is stored by our bodies in special fat cells. When food is not readily available and the body needs energy, fat is converted into fuel. This method of energy storage evolved over millions of years of human history and was vital to survival during lean periods when food sources were scarce.

In the ancient natural world, fat was very hard to come by. Seeds, nuts, plants, fish, and wild game were the only fat sources available. This factor, combined with an inconsistent and occasionally scarce food supply, forced nature to develop a strong connection between our sense of taste and our desire to eat foods that are good sources of fat. When humans began selecting foods based on taste, foods high in fat became the foods of choice. Think about the fatty foods available to us now, like fat-laden red meat from domesticated cattle or butter and cream from dairy cows. Those foods did not exist a thousand years ago and do not occur naturally in nature.

Sugar   Sugar is divided into two categories: complex carbohydrates and simple carbohydrates. Complex carbohydrates such as vegetables, fruits, and grains occur naturally. An example of a simple carbohydrate is white refined sugar. It is processed from sugarcane, and has no nutritional value other than to supply calories. Natural complex carbohydrates are the best sources of energy. Unlike simple carbohydrates, they metabolize slowly, providing a steady flow of fuel to keep us alert. Nature knew that. When we found this amazing energy fuel, we needed to eat it. Again, a strong connection between our sense of taste and a desire to eat carbohydrates developed.

Salt   Salt, the third major taste, is also crucial to our bodies. It maintains the balance of our body fluids, preventing dehydration by regulating key hormones. It helps the heart, the kidneys, and the adrenal glands to monitor all of our bodily functions. Salt helps maintain blood pressure and is necessary to the body's electrical system.

Salt occurs naturally in most foods, and it is those natural salts that our bodies crave and need. It is important to note that the organic salts found in plants and animals are not the same as table salt. The connection between taste and the desire to eat substances containing salt was established long ago in our brains. When preagricultural humans found organic substances that contained fat, sugar, and salt, their brains told them to eat and to eat a lot of the substances.

Through the process of evolution, survival of the human species depended on foods that possessed one or all of the three characteristics of taste. When we gained control of our food supply, we began to alter foods to satisfy our tastes. The foods we routinely choose to eat contain significantly more fat, sugar, and salt than occur naturally. Because our sense of taste and hunger connection is so strong, the concentration of fat, sugar, and salt in those foods increases dramatically.

What does all this mean? It simply means this: powerful biological mechanisms drive us to seek foods that are rich in fat, salt, and sugar and in our modern world, the foods that contain these substances are not what nature intended us to eat. These foods trick our bodies into believing they are receiving nutrition when most of the foods contain useless empty calories. As a result, it is this concentration of fat, sugar, and salt in the foods we eat that contributes to the increased occurrences of heart disease, cancer, hypertension, stroke, diabetes, kidney failure, and osteoporosis. The Surgeon General's Report on Nutrition and Health (1988) indicates that concerns about nutrition and health have expanded within recent years beyond the need to prevent deficiencies. In other words, our typical American diet is not only providing us with improper nutrition; it is killing us, slowly and insidiously.

The nutritionally related diseases of coronary heart disease, stroke, cancer, and diabetes are the leading causes of death and disability in the United States. Substantial scientific research over the past few decades indicates that diet can play an important role in preventing such conditions. Remember the expression, "you are what you eat." The only source of raw material for the cells in our bodies to replicate and continue life is contained in the foods we eat. Whether we realize it or not, what we put into our bodies in large measure determines the length and the quality of our lives.

Understanding this, we may surmise that our very lives depend on what we eat. A diet high in fat can clog our arteries and restrict the flow of blood to and from our hearts. Eventually our hearts are overworked and our cells do not receive the nutrition they need to function properly and renew themselves. We may then become one of the millions of people who suffer from coronary heart disease. Likewise, a diet high in refined sugar can lead to diabetes, obesity, kidney failure, depression, and cancer. For many people, too much salt can be deadly. Salt causes the body to retain excess water, and because the body can only hold a limited amount of fluid, the heart is strained tremendously. Excess salt can lead to kidney damage as well as a host of other complications.

CONSCIOUS DECISIONS

The key to a program of healing nutrition is making conscious efforts to eliminate or reduce foods that harm our bodies. No matter how hard we try to defend today's food choices, we must realize that most of these foods did not even exist 100 years ago. The truth is that our bodies are not really designed to eat these foods in the quantity that we do. The taste and hunger for fat, sugar, and salt in the Stone Age meant searching for food choices that would ensure survival. In the modern world, those same tastes and hungers led us to develop processed foods that are almost totally devoid of nutritional value but that taste good. Today we eat tons of great-tasting, lifeless food. For most of us, until it is too late, we never make the connection between the food we eat and how we feel physically.

In 1754, philosopher Jean Rousseau wrote that in a state of nature, men were strong of limb, fleet of foot, and clear of eye. Today, most of our ills are of our own making, and we might have avoided them by adhering to that simple manner of life prescribed by nature. The simple truth is that nature has provided us with all the basic means from which to build our bodies from birth to old age in a state of maximum health, to enjoy life experiences with abundant energy, vigor, and vitality, and to achieve a happy, long life span. The secret, which is really no secret at all, consists of making conscious decisions to put the right foods into our mouths at the right times. Only then will we have optimal nourishment and a proper state of mind. Right now, at the highest levels of government, our leaders are seeking ways to finance a system of health care that could cost a trillion dollars to treat all of the sick and dying citizens afflicted with the degenerative diseases of modern humans. Yet the cure for many of these ills is already available to us. It is not a miracle drug therapy, and it is not expensive. It is the food we eat and making the connection in our minds between the foods we eat today and the sickness and health that result years down the road.

Do no harm to your body. The meaning of that phrase seems obvious. People who care about their personal welfare would probably not intentionally do harm to their bodies. For example, would you stick your hand in a fire or walk into a street of oncoming traffic? These conscious acts are obviously potentially harmful to our bodies, but what about the potentially harmful things we do every day and never think about? Consider those unconscious acts we perform every time we sit down to eat. Doing no harm means we need to be consciously aware of any potential risk that could result from the kinds of foods we eat. It is not that we should never eat these foods, but that we should be conscious of what to eat daily. Strive to consciously limit those foods that contain excessive fat, sugar, and salt and to focus on foods that feed your cells super nutrition. An easy rule to remember is that before you put anything into your mouth, ask yourself one simple question—Will eating this food make my body feel good? Then make your choice about eating it based upon your answer.

When we walk into any modern supermarket we are faced with over 30,000 food choices. As we wheel our carts past the meat counter, the microwave section, through the canned food section, past the salty snack section, and past the dairy section, we end up in the produce aisle where most of our best food choices are located. Even the produce we choose today is not the same as that of our ancestors. It probably looks better because it has been polished and waxed. Remember that years of genetic engineering have gone into creating foods and vegetables that look good and have a long shelf life. Many of these foods are grown in mineral-deprived soils. Even though this produce looks perfect and tastes good, it is not the same as it once was 1,000 years ago.

We are faced with myriad food choices of which only a very small amount of foods are really any good for us. Many are either neutral or harmful. By paying a little closer attention to foods that are potentially harmful, we may be able to add significant quality years to our lives. It is important to remember that the foods to reduce are saturated fats, added salts, refined sugars, caffeine, and chemical additives. We will discuss each of these foods in the following chapters.

SUMMARY

The foods we put into our bodies affect how we look and feel and even impact our potential life spans. If you believe that the key to optimal health is the food that fuels our bodies, I invite you to continue to read about a new way of living that will increase your potential life span and help you to be increasingly healthy for the rest of your natural life.

References

Eat to live 120 years. (1992). Redmond, WA: Zygon International.

Pearson, D., & Shaw, S. (1982). *Life extension: A practical scientific approach.* New York: Warner Books.

U.S. Department of Health & Human Services. (1988). *The Surgeon General s report on nutrition and health.* DHHS (PHS) Publication No. 88-50211.

Willix, R. (1994). *3 minutes a day to a 120 year lifespan.* Baltimore, MD: Health for Life LLC.

3 FOOD AND DISEASE

The goal of healing nutrition is to maximize body-mind-spirit health. If we neglect nutritional self-care and add to the situation heredity and environmental factors, certainly disease and illness may occur. I group some of these beginning, non-life-threatening ailments into the category of "benign self-neglect." These seemingly benign disorders, if left unattended, have the potential to evolve into full-blown illnesses or diseases.

Detrimental nutritional states result from both undernutrition and overconsumption. Those who overconsume not only will be overweight, they may also be undernourished.

BENIGN SELF-NEGLECT

The concept of benign self-neglect is derived not because the outcomes are benign, but rather because the person who functions with a self-care deficit usually does so from an unaware or uninformed state of consciousness. We do not indulge in poor eating habits on purpose but rather because we do not know any better, have suppressed our knowledge in lieu of seemingly more important current events, or no longer have the motivation or desire for self-care. For example, the teenager with acne may be uninformed about the deleterious effects of junk food and inadequate skin hygiene. The young parent may be so busy chauffeuring, tutoring, and financing his child's rearing that he may, due to simple psychological overload, sit and eat chips, dips, candy, and sodas during his break without the kids. The fast track, upwardly mobile, career executive may believe that it is necessary to relax by having several drinks and a high-fat meal to unwind at the end of each busy workday. All of these individuals consciously think they are doing the best they can. The teen is concentrating on schoolwork, the parent on raising the children, and the executive on fulfilling career ambitions. None of them purposely mistreat their bodies. They are simply so busy concentrating on their lives' work that they fail to pause and consider the importance of good nutrition in their lives.

COMMON DISORDERS

The category of benign self-neglect includes a host of ailments. The ones most easily recognized are dental caries, fatigue, overweight, and constipation. These and other common disorders are detailed as follows:

Acne

The Problem   Acne is a disorder of the oil glands in the skin and is characterized by the recurring formation of blackheads, whiteheads, and pimples on the face and upper trunk. The incidence is greatest in puberty and adolescence when the hormones influencing the secretion of these specific oil glands are at their peak level of activity.

Interventions   Food choices during the teen years can affect the severity of the condition. A diet high in fat and refined sugars should be avoided. This means limiting intake of soft drinks, fried foods, desserts, and nuts. It has also been found that foods rich in oxalic acid, such as chocolate, spinach, and rhubarb, may inhibit the absorption of calcium. Because calcium is important in maintaining the acid-alkali balance of the blood, which is necessary for a clear complexion, these foods should be avoided if adolescent acne is a problem.

Vitamins A and B-complex are important to healthy, glowing skin. Both vitamins are often prescribed after the fact, so why wait? Encourage young people to eat foods high in these essential vitamins. Vitamin A clears the face while B-complex vitamins, especially riboflavin (B_2), pyridoxine (B_6), and pantothenic acid, help to reduce facial oiliness and blackhead formation.

Vitamins C, D, and E, and the mineral zinc also work to keep complexions healthy. Vitamin C aids in resisting the spread of infection while vitamin D safeguards the body's store of calcium from excretion. Vitamin E prevents scarring, while zinc is an effective bacterial suppressor. To see which foods will provide the vitamins and minerals discussed in this chapter, refer to chapter 8, tables 8.1 and 8.2.

Allergies

The Problem   Many people suffer from sensitivity to allergens. Allergens arise from pollens, molds, animal dander, chemicals, insect bites, and foods. Susceptibility to allergens is related to multiple factors, including heredity, stress, infections, and nutritional status. Healthy bodies are more likely to resist allergens, while inadequately nourished ones may possess weakened immune systems with increased cell permeability. This allows easy access to cell entrance by allergenic foreign substances.

Interventions   To combat allergies, the best method is to maintain a well-balanced healthy diet and avoid known allergens.

Body Odor

The Problem   External body odors are related to the internal health of the body.

Interventions   Certain nutrients seem to metabolically remove body wastes that cause odors. They include vitamins B_6 and PABA and the minerals magnesium and zinc.

Bruises

The Problem   Bruises are caused by the rupture of small blood vessels, resulting in discoloration of underlying tissues without a break in the overlying skin. Individuals who bruise easily, and have seen their health care practitioners to make certain they do not have diseases such as anemia or leukemia and do not use anticoagulants (like daily aspirin), should consider dietary factors.

Interventions   Vitamin C and the bioflavonoids strengthen the small blood vessels. Vitamin D is a natural blood-clotting agent. The antioxidants, vitamins A, C, E, B_1, B_5, and B_6, and the minerals zinc and selenium are also effective in combating the rupture of small vessels.

Bruxism (Teeth Grinding)

The Problem   The annoying condition of bruxism is one that most people think is beyond their control because it usually occurs during sleep. The unfortunate effects include enamel loss, gum recession, and awakening with a tight jaw.

Interventions   Although bruxism may be a condition that occurs primarily due to stress, certain vitamins and minerals may help. Calcium is effective for treating involuntary movements of muscles, while pantothenic acid aids in maintaining motor coordination. Both nutrients are also antistress formulas.

Colds

The Problem   The common cold is an annoying and always inconvenient occurrence. This highly contagious condition causes a general inflammation of the mucous membranes of the respiratory passages and is caused by a variety of viruses. The difficulty in curing the common cold is related to the multiple, constantly mutating viruses that are difficult to pinpoint.

Interventions   The best prevention of the common cold is to maintain the body at high nutritional and low stress levels. We should get adequate sleep and eat diets that invigorate the immune system. When a cold strikes, some vitamins are thought to be helpful. Vitamin B$_6$ is noted as a key vitamin that stimulates production of antibodies to defend the body against infection. Some authorities, the most notable being Linus Pauling, have considered vitamin C intake to be essential in both the prevention and treatment of colds. Prevention doses are from 1 to 2 grams daily, while as much as 600 to 625 milligrams every 3 hours (when awake) may be successful for treatment (Kirschmann, 1984).

Constipation

The Problem   Countless people suffer from the mostly unnecessary condition of constipation. This disorder is characterized by a decreased frequency of bowel movements resulting in waste matter remaining in the colon and becoming dry and difficult to expel.

Interventions   This condition, like many of the others, is related to simple body-mind-spirit behaviors. Constipation results from insufficient muscle tone in the bowel and/or abdominal wall that occurs due to poor habits. Lack of exercise, repeated failure to pay attention to and follow the body's signal to eliminate, insufficient fluid intake, or a diet lacking in roughage can all contribute to this disorder.

Food and body-mind training can prevent or correct this condition. Fruits, vegetables, and whole grains contain the high fiber necessary to create the needed bulk. Unsaturated fats are useful because they effectively lubricate the mucous walls of the colon. The allicin in garlic stimulates the walls of the intestines. Yogurt, buttermilk, and other milk products containing acidophilus cultures are beneficial in maintaining proper intestinal flora, especially during antibiotic therapy. Apples, papayas, pineapples, prunes, and figs also target intestinal motility. Needless to say, six to eight glasses of water (not teas, coffees, and sodas) are necessary to maintain adequate hydration.

Body-mind training is essential in this condition. Learning to heed the body's signal and discipline the system for a regular morning or start-of-day elimination time is part of curing this condition. Harmonizing the body with regular exercise is also essential to reverse or prevent constipation.

Dandruff

The Problem   Dandruff may be only dry flakes that occur when brushing hair or it may be a more serious condition, seborrheic dermatitis. Simple dandruff is the result of an inadequate diet and inefficient carbohydrate metabolism.

Interventions   Dandruff can usually be reversed with a diet of unrefined carbohydrates and B vitamins. The antioxidants, vitamins C and E, and the mineral selenium are also helpful (see chapter 8 for more information about antioxidants). Naturally, body-mind behaviors such as recognizing the need for a specialized shampoo and frequent washing and hair brushing are essential.

Dermatitis

The Problem   Dermatitis is an inflammatory, frequently recurring skin reaction. One form of dermatitis is eczema, an eruption of blisters on the skin that weep and crust. Itching, flaking, scaling, and eventual thickening and color changes of the skin may occur. This ailment, like the others, originates in body-mind-spirit behaviors. It may be associated with hereditary allergic traits and can be aggravated by stress and fatigue.

Interventions   If the irritant is a food item, it should be eliminated from the diet. Foods rich in the B vitamins have been found to cure infants who have dermatitis. Vitamin A is also essential for maintaining healthy skin.

Diarrhea

The Problem   Valuable vitamins and minerals can be lost through frequent, loose stools. Diarrhea can be caused by bacteria or viruses in contaminated food, emotional distress, food allergies, a diet too high in roughage, or overuse of laxatives or caffeine.

Interventions   When diarrhea occurs, supplement with vitamins C, B-complex, and sodium, magnesium, and potassium, which are lost through dehydration. Naturally, you want to take in copious fluids to replace the water lost through the stools.

Environmental Pollution

The Problem   We are continually exposed to pollutants in the air we breathe, the water we drink, and the food we eat. It is often years before the deleterious effects of these pollutants are realized. The results of these exposures range from birth defects to yellow teeth to plubism (lead poisoning).

Interventions   Some nutrients lessen the adverse effects of pollutants. The free radical scavengers, vitamins A, C, and E, provide some protection. Vitamin C also removes lead from bone and brain tissue, as well as prevents some of the carcinogenic nitrosamines from forming. Selenium has been found to protect against mercury poisoning.

Fatigue

The Problem   Who does not know what this means and how it feels? Unfortunately, it is all too often related to whole body health and, in large part, includes inadequate nutrition.

Interventions   The fast track to putting the zip back into your life includes formulating and following a balanced food program and daily movement regime. Correct deficiencies in B-complex, C, D, or iron to combat fatigue. The minerals magnesium and potassium may be supplemented to boost muscle strength.

Flatulence

The Problem   Lots of folks pass gas. The two most common causes are gulping air while eating and releasing of gases liberated by the putrefactive bacteria living on undigested food. Another cause is the deficiency of the enzyme lactose which assists in digesting milk products. During the aging process, enzyme production often decreases, causing flatulence to develop during the "graying" years. See chapter 10 for more information regarding enzyme supplements for aging.

Interventions   A diet of high-fiber foods, especially apples, cabbage, brussels sprouts, and beans will often induce flatulence due to the fibrous food remains fermenting in the intestines.

Pantothenic acid has been shown to relieve intestinal gas while the B vitamins aid in bowel motility. Yogurt and other milk products containing acidophilus bacillus aid in the digestion of high-fiber foods and replace friendly intestinal bacteria that may have been lost during diarrhea or destroyed during antibiotic therapy. Refer also to the use of herbs in chapter 13.

Hair Health

The Problem   Dull, thinning hair is no fun. Although heredity and age play a significant role in hair loss, hair quality is, in fact, related to nutrition.

Interventions   Protein deficiency affects hair color, texture, and quantity. When protein intake is boosted, hair quality often improves. Vitamins A, B_6, biotin, and folic acid are also essential for healthy hair. Women who use birth control pills (BCP) or are in their last months of pregnancy sometimes experience hair loss. This may be attributed to an imbalance of copper. The hair regrows following delivery or when the BCPs are switched or discontinued.

Halitosis

The Problem   Bad breath can be caused by improper diet, respiratory infections, poor oral hygiene, alcohol intake, or smoking. In some cases, it may be related to ingested chemicals such as arsenic, lead, bismuth, or methane. Even nervous tension can be the cause, but it is usually attributed to expulsion of gas from putrefactive bacteria through the mouth.

Interventions   In addition to proper oral hygiene, a carefully regulated diet is essential to combat this socially disastrous disorder. Vitamin C is necessary to ensure oral health and prevent scurvy, while vitamin A is needed for the overall development and robust maintenance of the gums and teeth.

Headache

The Problem Headaches may be one of the most annoying manifestations of benign self-neglect. Tension headaches result from contractions of the neck, scalp, or forehead muscles; vascular headaches come from uneven dilation of cerebral vessels; and sinus headaches are caused by inflamed mucous membranes of the sinus cavities, causing misery to millions on a daily basis.

Interventions There certainly are pathogenic and hereditary factors that cause this ailment, but most headaches can be soothed, abated, and even eliminated by a long-term course of body-mind-spirit therapies. A full gamut of stress reduction therapies supplemented by a farsighted nutrition therapy program can break the headache cycle. The B-complex vitamins, especially niacin, are important in maintaining normal dilation of the cerebral blood vessels. Iron, pantothenic acid, and vitamin A have proved helpful to some people. The minerals calcium, zinc, magnesium, and potassium and the amino acid tryptophan have helped migraine sufferers. Acidophilus establishes and maintains the proper intestinal bacteria from which the body self-produces the B vitamins.

Hemorrhoids

The Problem These ruptured or distended veins located around the ring of the anus are unseen but felt by the sufferer. Hemorrhoids can be caused by improper lifting or by pregnancy, but more often than not, they are caused by lifestyle and nutritional factors. Diets too low in roughage and water and too high in slow-moving fats and protein foods play a major role. Poor diet, a sedentary life, and excess body weight can be common causes for a case of the "piles."

Interventions Hemorrhoids can be avoided and in some cases completely reversed with proper nutrition, exercise, hygiene, weight management, and improved elimination patterns. Dietary intake should include high-fiber foods, six to eight glasses of water per day, and the Recommended Daily Allowances (RDAs) of vitamins A, C, E, and B-complex.

Indigestion

The Problem   Dyspepsia is incomplete digestion that manifests in the symptoms of distension, heartburn, abdominal cramps, gas, and occasional nausea. Although it can sometimes be attributed to bacterial contamination of food, it is frequently the result of what and how we eat. Overeating, gulping air with meals, or eating during times of psychological distress can induce dyspepsia. Smoking during meals or overconsumption of gastric irritants such as coffee, tea, chocolate, or alcohol are also causative factors. Drinking copious quantities of fluids immediately before or while eating can cause indigestion. Too much fluid around mealtimes can wash the essential hydrochloric acid out of the stomach and result in decreased digestive enzymes, which are necessary to digest the food.

Interventions   How you eat is important in this condition. Eat slowly, drink minimally during meals, and chew thoroughly while ingesting healing foods. Wait until you are in or induce a joyful state of mind-spirit before beginning your meal. Papaya or its commercial extract contains one of the important enzymes that aids in protein digestion in the stomach. An herbal peppermint tea can also soothe the digestive tract and stimulate digestive secretions.

Leg Cramps

The Problem   Involuntary spasms of muscles in the leg or foot most commonly occur at night and are most frequent in the young, elderly, and persons with arteriosclerosis. In the case of the elder with arteriosclerosis, it is difficult to alleviate leg cramps without surgery. In the absence of arteriosclerosis, the most common cause of leg cramps is a calcium deficiency. In some cases, a sodium loss incurred through heavy perspiration or diarrhea may be the causative factor.

Interventions   The RDAs for vitamins B, C, and B-complex should be followed to maintain muscle strength. In addition, sufficient quantities of the minerals calcium, magnesium, and sodium need to be maintained. Remember, too, that protein rebuilds damaged tissues.

Nail Problems

The Problem Unhealthy fingernails or toenails may be the result of local injury, pathophysiology, or nutrient deficiency. Because nails are composed almost entirely of protein, suspect this area of the diet first.

Interventions Dietary treatment includes protein and vitamins A and B-complex. B-complex deficiencies result in fragile nails with horizontal or vertical ridges. Lack of vitamin A or calcium can cause dryness or brittleness. Frequent hangnails indicate inadequate quantities of vitamin C, folic acid, and protein. Nailbed white spots indicate zinc deficiency.

Overweight and Obesity

The Problem Fifty percent of American adults and 25 percent of the country's teenagers are overweight. This reversible condition contributes to all the major illnesses, including heart disease, diabetes, kidney disorders, and psychological problems. Few people, if any, are overweight on purpose. This is indeed a disorder of benign self-neglect.

Interventions This malady can be corrected by conscious awakening and attending to one's body-mind-spirit needs. Refer to chapter 18 for more information on this topic.

Stress

The Problem The increased production of adrenal hormones that occurs with stress increases the metabolism of protein, fats, and carbohydrates necessary to produce instant energy for the body to use to combat the perceived stressor. As a result of this increased metabolism, there is also an increased excretion of the minerals potassium, phosphorus, and calcium. Vitamin C is used by the adrenals, so if the stress is sufficiently severe or prolonged, there will be a depletion of this vitamin in the tissues. Many of the disorders related to stress are not the result of the stressor itself, but rather a result of nutritional deficiencies caused by increased metabolic rate during this period of time.

Interventions If you are experiencing stress, you must pay special attention to a well-balanced diet and emphasize replacing the nutrients and vitamins depleted during this time.

Tics, Tremors, and Twitches

The Problem These potentially embarrassing disorders may result from ineffective coping with stress or they may be directly related to an imbalance of minerals in the body. The most common cause is a deficiency of potassium and/or magnesium. These minerals are essential for the conduction of nerve impulses that pass to a muscle and control its movement. Sometimes the B-complex vitamins, which are related to health of the nervous system, are found to be deficient. When the deficiency is corrected with supplements or B-rich foods, the symptoms may disappear. Twitches are occasionally caused by an increase of lead in the body or an allergic reaction to an allergen. If excessive lead is discovered, an intake of calcium or zinc can effectively leach the toxic metal out of the body.

Tooth and Gum Disorders

The Problem Dental caries can ruin an otherwise pretty smile. Most cavities are caused by persistent eating of refined sugars and starches that, when mixed with saliva, form an acid that erodes tooth enamel. Although cavities are the major dental disease, periodontitis is the ailment that causes the loss of teeth. This condition begins with gingivitis in which the gums swell, redden, and tend to bleed. Left untreated, this can lead to pyorrhea, which is characterized by further gum inflammation, recession, and loosening of teeth.

Interventions To prevent this condition, you must practice proper oral hygiene and eat right. All vitamins and minerals are essential with vitamins A and C being critical. Vitamin A regulates the development and general health of the gums, while vitamin C is important for the maintenance of healthy gums. The minerals sodium, potassium, calcium, phosphorus, iron, and magnesium are also needed.

The preceding ailments are a sampling of what can happen when we become so busy that we forget to take care of ourselves. The positive aspect of this issue is that most of these conditions can be reversed with conscientious nutritional self-care.

ILLNESS AND DISEASE

How fortunate we are in the 1990s to understand many of the truths concerning the relationship between nutrition and disease. Today it seems hard to believe it was only a couple of generations ago that Americans suffered from debilitating diseases such as rickets, beriberi, pellagra, and scurvy. Thanks to nutritional researchers who unraveled these axioms, these gross-deficiency diseases are now understood, and because we know they can be prevented with food, these diseases are rarely found today. This is not to say, however, that these nutritional diseases have been eradicated. Unfortunately, inhabitants in many Third World countries and some Americans still succumb to the ravages of these maladies.

People in developed nations may not have kwashiorkor or have their teeth fall out because of scurvy, but that does not mean that we do not suffer from other, less obvious effects of deficient diets. Actually, very few of us are as vibrantly healthy as we might be. About one-third of us will develop heart disease and one in five will die of cancer. Millions of us require medication for anxiety, depression, or pain to suppress or control the ravages of chronic diseases. Three out of 10 women will develop osteoporosis after menopause, while some 40 percent of men will develop prostate trouble. Although we may feel well enough to function and meet basic needs, we may be one of the masses who is on the borderline when it comes to living a truly healthy lifestyle.

The more we learn about the fascinating science of nutrition the more we begin to understand the incredibly important relationship between what we eat and how we feel. The following list depicts diseases that are still with us, some of which are on the increase. Each of the ailments may be categorized as a major disease and each of them is in some way related to nutrition. Overall well-being can be helped by an adequate diet for sufferers of these diseases. The important concept to understand is that each of these diseases can be positively affected by nutritional realignment.

Alcoholism	Hypertension
Anemia	Intestinal parasites
Arteriosclerosis and athero-sclerosis	Kidney diseases and renal stones
Arthritis	Mental illness
Asthma	Mononucleosis
Bronchitis	Neuritis
Bursitis	Osteoporosis
Cancer	Pancreatitis
Cataracts	Parkinson's disease
Celiac disease	Pellagra
Cirrhosis	Pernicious anemia
Colitis	Phlebitis
Conjunctivitis	Pneumonia
Cystitis	Polio
Diabetes	Psoriasis
Diverticulitis	Pyorrhea
Decubiti	Rheumatic fever
Gallstones	Rheumatism
Gastritis	Rickets
Glaucoma	Sciatica
Gout	Scurvy
Heart disease	Shingles (herpes zoster)
Hepatitis	Sinusitis
Herpes Simplex	

SUMMARY

Nurses have the opportunity to awaken those persons with whom they come in contact in their day-to-day practices. We have the ability to empower masses of people to recognize that how, what, where, why, with whom, and when we eat makes a difference in our lives. However, we must first care for ourselves to become walking, talking, living examples of vibrant health. Only then will we be in fit condition to lead others.

Part 2 of this text offers a guide for understanding the basics of nutrition. These scientific facts and figures provide us with the data we need to function as knowledgeable nurse-healers.

Reference

Kirschmann, J. (1984). *Nutrition almanac.* New York: McGraw-Hill Book Co.

Part

2 UNDERSTANDING THE BASICS

4 BASIC NUTRITIONAL NEEDS

It is elevating to think of our bodies as temples for our souls. Temples, like ordinary buildings, require continual attention to ensure firm, long-standing, vital structures. In order to build and maintain strong, resilient frames in which to house our souls, we should know about our bodies' fundamental needs and how best to meet them. Human organisms are collections of bones, muscles, organs, tissues, and cells. All of these structures are composed of chemicals that come directly from the foods we eat. Human beings are remarkable creatures endowed with physical, mental, and spiritual properties that can only be actualized by an adequate intake of nourishment. The nourishment we need is multifaceted, but it includes the nutritional intake of the earth's good foods. Figure 4.1 depicts the composition of the human body in terms of chemical nutrients.

NUTRITIONAL TERMS

Some of the most common nutritional terms are defined as follows:

> *Nutrition*—the process by which living things utilize food for energy, growth, development, and maintenance. We

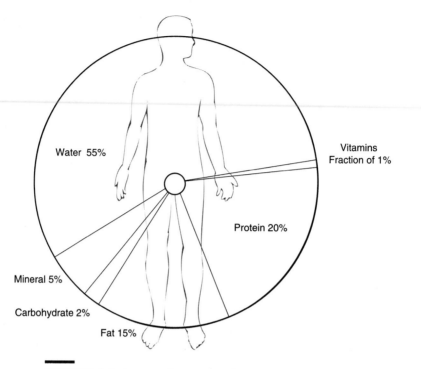

Water 55%

Vitamins
Fraction of 1%

Protein 20%

Mineral 5%

Carbohydrate 2%

Fat 15%

FIGURE 4.1 Approximate nutrient composition of the human body.

eat foods to provide nutrients for necessary body functions and to make essential compounds. Many of these nutrients cannot be synthesized, so we must obtain them in our daily food. Nutrition involves digesting foods and absorbing and delivering nutrients to the cells where they are utilized. It also includes picking up and carrying the waste products to the bloodstream.

Food—any substance ingested into the body to provide nutrients.

Gram—a unit of weight. Most food labels list contents in terms of grams. For many foods, 30 grams equals 1 ounce.

Health—the state of optimal physical, mental, spiritual, and social well-being.

Nutrients—biochemical substances used by the body. The six major classes of nutrients obtained from foods are water, protein, carbohydrates, fats, minerals, and vitamins.

Malnutrition—a condition that arises from a prolonged lack of or excessive intake of nutrients or an impaired utilization of food.

Megadose—a quantity of a vitamin or mineral that exceeds by 10 times or more the RDA of that substance.

Recommended Dietary Allowances (RDAs)—identify nutritional needs in terms of specific amounts of nutrients that a healthy individual should receive every day. These nutrients help us achieve full growth and development potential. RDAs were intended to be desirable daily amounts of nutrients to be consumed by healthy people. This term was introduced in 1973 as a reference value for vitamins, minerals, and protein in voluntary nutritional labeling. In 1992, the term was renamed Reference Daily Intakes (RDIs). Despite the name change, the actual values (except for the value of protein) remains the same.

Daily Reference Values (DRVs)—figures for nutrients such as fat and cholesterol for which no standards previously existed. The figures are based on the number of calories consumed per day. For labeling purposes, 2,000 calories has been established as the reference for calculating percent daily values. Whatever the caloric level, DRVs for the energy-producing nutrients are always calculated as follows:

- Fat based on 30 percent of calories
- Saturated fat based on 10 percent of calories
- Carbohydrates based on 60 percent of calories
- Protein based on 10 percent of calories
- Fiber based on 11.5 grams of fiber per 1,000 calories

The DRVs for cholesterol, sodium, and potassium, which do not contribute calories, remain the same regardless of the calorie level. Table 4.1 shows DRVs of the major food components.

Food Component	DRV
Fat	65 grams
Saturated fatty acids	20 grams
Cholesterol	300 milligrams
Total carbohydrate	300 grams
Fiber	25 grams
Sodium	2,400 milligrams
Potassium	3,500 milligrams
Protein**	50 grams

*Based on 2,000 calories a day for adults and children over 4 years old

**DRV for protein does not apply to certain populations; Reference Daily Intake (RDI) for protein has been established for these groups: children 1 to 4 years: 16 grams; infants under a year: 14 grams; pregnant women: 60 grams; and nursing women: 65 grams.

Source: *FDA Consumer*, May 1993

TABLE 4.1   Daily Reference Values (DRVs)*

WATER AND CHEMICALS

Water

Cosmic dust swirled from the universe and settled in the Milky Way Galaxy billions of years ago to form planet Earth. Water, the liquid from which life arose, was probably locked into rock-forming compounds. These compounds slowly released the trapped water during the first billion years or so of Earth's history and formed the primordial oceans. Water became the most common substance on Earth and now covers more than 70 percent of the planet's surface. From the primordial saline oceans, living, breathing organisms arose, and from those organisms came human life. All living things consist mostly of water; our bodies are about two-thirds water. Because so much of our physical being is fluid, we need to keep recycling our systems with clean, fresh water. We are advised to drink six to eight glasses of pure water each day because we need to continually renew our body fluids.

Just as the ocean provides tremendous means of transportation for the cargo of goods distributed worldwide, the fluid in our arteries and veins serves as the transportation system for the whole of our bodies. Oceans clearly play an essential role in life on Earth, yet because of their vastness, humans have used their waters as dumping grounds for many waste materials. Just as we must not allow our oceans to become polluted, so too we must keep our bodies clean by replenishing them with clean, pure water. Waste materials and toxins need daily flushings to maintain homeostasis. Homeostasis, which is standard for any healthy organism, involves the maintenance of a steady state within a biological system by means of self-regulating mechanisms.

Chemical Composition

The human body is made up of numerous chemical elements, but the main components are oxygen, hydrogen, carbon, and nitrogen. These elements, which are derived directly or indirectly from the atmosphere or from water, account for nearly 95 percent of total body weight. The remaining elements include:

1. The minerals calcium and phosphorus, which as constituents of bone account for about another 3 percent of body weight

2. In order of decreasing amounts: potassium, sodium, magnesium, iron, zinc, and copper

3. Several trace elements such as vanadium, chromium, silicon, and selenium

On the molecular level, the body's chemicals are organized into two major categories: inorganic and organic compounds. Organic compounds are the carbon-containing compounds, the main types of which include proteins, lipids, and carbohydrates. Each of these compounds is discussed in detail in other chapters. Water constitutes roughly 60 percent of total body weight and is essential for almost all chemical reactions within the body.

The molecular constituents of the body are combined to form cells and extracellular materials. The adult human body contains approximately 100 trillion cells, which are organized and differentiated to form a number of different kinds of tissues with specific functions. We can affect these trillions of cells with healing nutrition. Since we are constantly shedding old cells and developing new ones, we have the opportunity to build new cells with the best nutritional elements and compounds available.

It is from our cells that we build the four main types of tissue: epithelial, muscle, nerve, and connective. Epithelial tissue, which covers the body's surface and lines its tubes, protects these surfaces. Epithelial tissue is the site of various absorption and excretion processes. Also included in epithelial tissue are the outgrowths and ingrowths that form the surfaces of sensory organs, glands, hair, nails, and other structures. Muscle tissue provides movement to the body through its ability to contract and relax. Nerve tissue, made up of neurons, conducts information signals and processes data. Connective tissue, which contains large amounts of extracellular matter, provides support for the body in the form of tendons, ligaments, cartilage, bone, and fat deposits. Lastly, blood and lymph are fluids that are sometimes also considered as tissues. Together they convey nutrients, waste products, and the specialized defensive cells of the immune system through the different parts of the body.

CALORIC REQUIREMENTS

For the most part, we Americans consume more calories than we need. Caloric requirements depend on your size, age, and level of activity. Table 4.2 denotes some approximate daily caloric needs.

Number of calories	Body Type, Age, and Level of Activity
1,600	sedentary women
	some older adults
2,200	most children
	teenage girls
	active women (pregnant or lactating women may need more)
	sedentary men
2,800	teenage boys
	most active men
	very active women
3,000 and up	athletes in training

TABLE 4.2   Basic Caloric Requirements

Foods vary markedly in their caloric values. When attempting to stay within a range of caloric consumption, it is important to know which foods will add substantial calories to our intake.

Table 4.3 lists common foods and the calories they provide.

Item	Amount	Calories
Cottage cheese	1 cup	225
Mozzarella	1 ounce	90
American cheese	1 ounce	105
Sour cream	1 cup	230
Yogurt (flavored, whole milk)	1 cup	260
Yogurt (skim milk)	1 cup	127
Boiled egg	1	80
Fried egg	1	85
Butter	1 stick	865
Fish (baked)	3 ounces	135
Crab meat	1 cup	135
Tuna meat (oil packed)	1 cup	295
Tuna meat (water packed)	1 cup	160
Bacon	2 slices	85
Beef (very lean)	3 ounces	245
Ham (lean)	3 ounces	245
Chicken breast	2.8 ounces	160
Apple	1	80
Avocado	1	370
Banana	1	100
Bread	1 loaf	1,195
Bread	1 slice	65
Chocolate chip cookies	4	200
Macaroni and cheese	1 cup	430
Walnuts	1 cup	785
Green beans (frozen)	1 cup	35
Corn (frozen)	1 cup	134

TABLE 4.3   *Caloric Content of Common Foods*

DIETARY FIBER

Dietary fiber includes all food substances that our digestive enzymes cannot break down. Since we cannot digest fiber, it is not used by the body as an energy source. There are six major types of dietary fiber:

- Cellulose—the major constituent of plant fiber, found in the plant cell walls

- Hemicellulose—closely associated with the cell walls of plants

- Lignin—the woody compound found not only in wood but also in plant fibers

- Pectin—substance found in roots, stems, and fruits of plants, especially in apples and citrus rinds; famous for its jelling properties

- Gums and mucilage—occur naturally in foods such as guar and legumes, and are used in many prepared food products

- Algal polysaccharides—found in sea vegetables; include kelp, kombu, carrageenan, and agar; these are gel-forming fibers

Each of the six types of fibers fit into one of two basic categories: water insoluble (which do not dissolve in water) and water soluble (which mix with water). Insoluble fibers such as those found in cellulose, hemicellulose, and lignin stimulate the intestines, decrease food transit time, and increase the weight and softness of the stool. Insoluble fiber is found in bran, whole grains, fruits, vegetables, and nuts.

The soluble fibers of pectin, gums, mucilages, algal polysaccharides, and certain hemicelluloses are found in fruits, oats, barley, legumes, psyllium, seeds, flax seeds, and sea vegetables. Responsible for most beneficial effects of fiber, these soluble fibers lower the absorption of cholesterol, regulate the blood sugar by slowing the absorption of sugar into the bloodstream, and absorb and remove toxic materials and carcinogens from the body. Although they are important to all of us, soluble fibers are of special interest to individuals with diabetes because these fibers keep the blood sugar at a more constant level. Hypoglycemia may be treated by using the slow sugar absorption properties of soluble fibers. Insoluble fibers, however, do not stabilize the blood sugar in the same way.

Wheat bran is one of the least expensive ways to obtain insoluble fiber. Wheat bran is easily added to breads, casseroles, soups, and cereals. Because it is extremely high in insoluble fibers, wheat bran accelerates transit time more than most foods by acting as an irritant to the intestines. Wheat bran must be used with large amounts of water to prevent cramping, flatulence, or constipation. Unlike soluble fibers, wheat bran increases the absorption rate of sugars into the bloodstream which may cause adverse blood sugar fluctuations in hypoglycemic and diabetic conditions. Since it is high in mineral-binding phytic acid, which binds minerals and makes them unavailable for the body to absorb, wheat bran should be used in moderation.

Oat bran, an excellent soluble fiber noted for its use in lowering cholesterol, is as effective as other soluble fibers. Like wheat bran, oat bran can be added to breads, casseroles, soups, and cereals, or it can be made into a cooked cereal. Its lighter color, texture, and flavor make it even more appealing than wheat bran. Since it contains some natural oils, it should be refrigerated or stored in the freezer for no more than two months.

Flax seeds are most commonly used as a healthy addition to breads and baked goods. The outer walls of the seeds swell and absorb water to form a mucilage coating that provides bulk and lubrication.

Guar gum, which is often found listed on the labels of commercially prepared whipped cream products, is a mucilaginous substance derived from legumes. Guar gum acts in a similar fashion to pectin.

Pectin, which is found in apples, is purified and used in antidiarrhea preparations. It is also used when making jams and jellies. It forms a jellylike substance and has all the beneficial effects of other soluble fibers.

Psyllium seeds are similar to flax seeds and are derived from the plantago plant. Most are used for their fiber-rich husks. The outer walls of the seeds swell and absorb water to form a mucilage coating that provides bulk and lubrication. Because psyllium seeds swell so rapidly, preparations made with them should be used immediately. Psyllium seeds have been used in many commercial laxatives for years.

How Much Fiber Do We Need?

The average low-fiber, refined diet provides about 10 to 20 grams of fiber per day. Conservative recommended daily intake quantity is 25 to 35 grams per day, but suggested optimal amounts range from 30 to 50 grams per day. Any increase should be gradual in order to give the digestive system time to adjust. The amount of water taken in needs to be increased as well.

To increase fiber intake, start by eating a bran muffin instead of a croissant and brown rice instead of white rice. Do

not peel vegetables unless they are waxed or have suffered surface damage, but be sure to wash them thoroughly. Eat whole
fruit instead of drinking the juice. Generally, counting grams of
fiber is not necessary if high-fiber substitutions are made. When
reading food tables and labels, look for the words *dietary fiber*
instead of *crude fiber*. Dietary fiber includes all the different
fibers present in a food.

Adjusting to Increased Fiber

Increasing fiber intake may cause:

- Digestive discomforts. Common reactions to increased
  fiber in the diet are flatulence and bloating. However,
  both can be minimized if proper precautions are taken.
  Gradually increasing fiber intake will decrease these
  symptoms. This means adding just one serving of a
  high-fiber food daily for a week. The next week, add
  another serving per day. Make ongoing diet changes
  that include high-fiber foods rather than processed, low-
  fiber foods. The second important step is to increase
  liquid intake to about 8 to 10 glasses of water per day
  to account for the extra liquid that will be absorbed by
  the fiber. This is the real key for the effectiveness of
  fiber. Too little liquid combined with more fiber intake
  can cause constipation.

- Mineral deficiencies. Too much fiber may lead to mineral deficiencies because fiber compounds, especially
  phytic acid and oxalic acid, bind with minerals to block
  absorption. However, mineral-binding phytic acid can
  be destroyed if high-fiber grains, nuts, and legumes are
  cooked, fermented, sprouted, or made into a yeast-
  risen bread.

- Changes in the body's use of medications in certain
  illnesses. Individuals with specific medical conditions,
  especially diabetes, hypoglycemia, and elevated cholesterol, should discuss an increase in fiber with their
  doctor, dietitian, or qualified health professional.
  Increased fiber may reduce the need for insulin and
  other medications.

High-Fiber Foods

Since all fiber sources except lignin are complex carbohydrates, the best way to increase fiber in the diet is to eat whole foods that are high in complex carbohydrates. Overprocessed foods like white flour, white sugar, and white rice are low in fiber and in other nutrients. Canned fruits and vegetables are much lower in fiber than their fresh whole or frozen counterparts. Overcooking also reduces the amount of available fiber. Try to include both insoluble and soluble fibers in your diet. Table 4.4 details the fiber content of some foods.

Food	Serving	Grams of Dietary Fiber
Whole wheat bread	1 slice	2.6
White bread	1 slice	0.63
Granola	1/2 cup	6.4
Oatmeal	1/2 cup, cooked	2.1
Popcorn	1 cup	1.3
Brown rice	1/2 cup, cooked	3.7
White rice	1/2 cup, cooked	1.5
Black beans	1/2 cup, cooked	7.7
Almonds	1/4 cup, whole	4.4
Broccoli	1/2 cup, cooked	5.5
Carrot	1 medium, raw	2.3
Kale (without stems)	1 cup, cooked	3.5
Lettuce (loose leaf)	1 cup, chopped	0.8
Peas, frozen	1/2 cup, cooked	3.6
Potato (med.)	1 baked in peel	4.7
Winter squash	1 cup, baked	6.9
Apple	1 medium	3.5
Banana	1 fresh	2.3
Figs	2 medium, dried	4.0
Orange	1 medium	3.1
Orange juice	1 cup, fresh	1.0
Peach	1 medium	1.5

TABLE 4.4   Fiber Content in Selected Foods

NURSING ROLES REGARDING NUTRITION

To be effective nurses, we need to know facts and figures to support our scientific knowledge base. Despite the power of data and numbers, we need more. As human beings striving to actualize our human potentials and helping others reach theirs, we need information that stimulates our motivation, stirs our psyche, and awakens our dreams. For many, it is the hope or dream of a better life or release from the clutches of illness or disease that motivates change. Nurses encounter clients in every conceivable life circumstance. It is nurses, armed with nutrition information and knowledge of how to stimulate motivation for lifestyle change, who can help clients realize the power of healthy nutrition. Specific clinical roles include counseling or guidance in the following areas:

- Lifestyle behavioral changes

- General nutrition

- Eating disorders

- Special clinical diets: diabetes, cancer, and heart disease

- Maternal, child, and elder nutrition

- Weight reduction and weight management programs

Teamwork is effective in many areas of healing; nutrition is no exception. When providing guidance to clients, rely on the help and support of nutritionists and other healing professionals.

FOOD MISINFORMATION

It is important to note that although traditional nutrition, like "traditional" everything else, is undergoing revolution, there is still much valuable information in our basic textbooks. Although this book includes some otherwise scantly covered information such as living foods and vegetarianism, it does not negate the adequacy of numerous basic nutrition guides. When studying nutrition, it is important not to fall prey to food faddist claims of panaceas. Characteristics of food faddists may be that they include one or more of the following arguments in their conversations:

1. Only certain foods will cure your condition

2. Certain foods are harmful and should be eliminated from your diet

3. Particular food combinations have special therapeutic effects

4. You may be vitamin or mineral deficient if you do not measure up to their muscle-testing method

5. Only natural foods or vitamins can meet nutritional needs and prevent disease

All or any one of these claims should make you suspicious. Healthy nutrition is not about eliminating or adding any one product to your diet. It is about discovering and maintaining balance with all food groups as you simultaneously balance your mind and spirit.

Unscientific information about food can mislead you and your clients and contribute to poor food habits and a rapidly emptying pocketbook. False information may be based on subtle half-truths, innuendos, or outright deception. Food faddists appeal to vulnerable groups such as the elderly and overweight people. Figure-conscious people or those with an exaggerated idea of glamour can fall prey to flashy advertisements that offer crash programs to achieve the ideal weight, muscle strength, beauty, or vitality. The best protection against food charlatans is to augment your knowledge of healing nutrition. Practice it and teach it to your clients. Remember, as much as we have come to respect our intuitive abilities, nursing is based in science. When clients ask us to evaluate a nutritional program, we need to teach them the value of asking significant questions. They, in turn, should ask these questions of diet or food promoters.

1. What is the program about?

2. What is the rationale for the program?

3. What is your evidence?

4. How does it work?

CASE STUDY | *Elizabeth*

Elizabeth was a 17-year-old high school junior. She struggled to be a high achiever and studied conscientiously for her finals and for the Scholastic Aptitude Test (SAT).

She knew that if she could maintain her 3.6 grade point average (GPA), and score over 1,200 on the SAT, she would be eligible for a college scholarship that could make all the difference in her life.

Elizabeth was first seen at the end of June by a health professional at one of the city emergency rooms. Her primary complaint was that her mouth was sore and her gums were bleeding. She had a temperature of 101°F and felt tired and listless. The young doctor in the emergency room told her she probably had some sort of virus but prescribed antibiotics just in case it was a bacterial infection. Three days later, when she felt no better and her teeth began to feel loose, her mother took her to a nurse practitioner who had special evening clinic sessions at the high school.

When the nurse questioned Elizabeth about dietary intake, she learned that in addition to being under tremendous stress regarding her academic achievement, Elizabeth was dieting. Elizabeth had lost 20 pounds during the past 6 weeks and intended to shed 10 more. She thought she had gained entirely too much weight during the academic year. Now that the school year was over, she had put her books aside, was concentrating on weight loss, and was helping her mother move out of their home into an apartment. When the nurse asked Elizabeth, "Do you think you may be under some stress?" the reply was immediate, "Of course I am! I never have a free minute and I worry about our new living arrangements all the time. Wouldn't you be under stress too?" In response to questions about her diet, Elizabeth said she primarily ate chicken noodle soup with occasional dill pickles for snacks. That diet had worked for some of her friends and she suspected that it would work for her too. Besides, she had heard that chicken soup was supposed to be healing.

The nurse thought Elizabeth was probably severely nutritionally deficient and counseled her and her mother about dietary recommendations. She also gave Elizabeth a pamphlet on stress management and referred her to a local dentist.

The dentist made the final diagnosis of scurvy. He debrided Elizabeth's mouth with pressure sprays of grapefruit juice and gave her prescriptions for lysine, vitamin C, and acidophilis. He reinforced the nurse's instructions for long periods of rest and relaxation as he told Elizabeth and her mother that she had a disease of stress. The emotional pressure she had been under for months had undermined her vitamin C stores. Because she was dieting and not eating fruits and vegetables or taking vitamin supplements, she had no vitamin C intake. She also did not have sufficient intake of the essential amino acids to rebuild new tissues and hence developed one of humankind's oldest ailments.

Elizabeth and her mother were amazed that she had come so close to actually losing her teeth because of misguided and insufficient nutritional information. After that experience, both mother and daughter became converts to balanced nutritional eating patterns.

Observations

Elizabeth was misdiagnosed and undertreated in the hospital emergency room because the physician did not consider nutrition as a possible cause of disease. People in good nutritional health are usually robust with bright eyes and shiny hair. Fatness or thinness is not an indication of nutritional health. Elizabeth deviated radically from healthy nutritional guidelines. When doing physical examinations and taking histories, we must remember that nutrition continues to be an important part of the overall health assessment.

SUMMARY

Good nutrition is an essential part of life. Without attention to what we eat, we have the unfortunate potential to develop both acute and/or chronic problems.

5 | PROTEINS

COMPOSITION

Proteins, the main building blocks of cells, are large, complex molecules (macromolecules) made up of polypeptides, which in turn are made up of the nitrogen-containing amino acids. Proteins constitute about 15 percent of the body by weight, form much of the body's structure, and serve important chemical functions, particularly in the form of enzymes. Proteins are essential molecules that people must have to maintain the structure and function of a healthy body. They have many different properties and function in a variety of ways. The term *protein* is derived from the Greek word *proteios*, meaning "primary." Enzymes, hemoglobin, certain hormones, and the collagen in bones, tendons, and skin are all proteins.

Proteins exist in diverse, complex structures that specify their particular function. The group is comprised of about 20 amino acids. Each amino acid is composed of an amino group, a carboxyl group, and a carbon side chain which specifies the characteristics of the particular amino acid. A primary protein is simply a long chain of amino acids linked together with a peptide bond between the amino group of one and the carboxyl group of another. The sequence of the amino acids in the chain varies with each type of protein. The amino acids constituting a protein are arranged in such a way as to give rise to periodic, secondary structures. The way in which a protein folds into its final conformation, or shape, is vital to its function.

CASE STUDY | *Cynthia*

Cynthia was a 19-year-old generic nursing student who was determined to look good and feel fit as she studied to become a nurse. When she entered the program a year ago, she saw that many of her student peers and practicing nurses were overweight and she resolved not to allow this to happen to her. She began an unmonitored, self-imposed, protein-restricted diet and remained on it for a year. She did stay slim, but as she entered her sophomore year, she began to notice some physical changes. Her hair lost its luster, her fingernails broke, and she felt tired all the time.

In her sophomore year, Cynthia took a required nutrition course. While taking this course, she learned the important role of food in health and realized that she had the symptoms of protein deficiency. She quickly modified her food intake to include adequate proteins. Within three months, her symptoms reversed and her energy returned. Cynthia was lucky. Others who are unaware of or do not realize the significance of healing nutrition can succumb to multiple diseases of omission or even premature death.

Observations

Unfortunately, Cynthia is typical of many young girls. In an effort to look svelte and be popular, many teenagers and young women sacrifice good nutrition for poor health. Lack of protein can cause patchy brown spots to appear on the skin and loss of hair. It can instigate diarrhea, anemia, vitamin deficiencies, fluid retention, and high blood pressure. Mental problems can also result from the lack of protein. Clients may experience maladies such as apathy, irritability, poor concentration, memory loss, and general fatigue. As nurses, we need to be alert to problems of faulty nutrition in people.

PROTEIN AND DIET

Protein is a critically important part of the diet. While plants synthesize all the amino acids required for building the necessary proteins, animals do not. Humans need dietary intake to synthesize eight essential amino acids, and therefore, are dependent on food to maintain health. Proteins help replace and form new tissue and transport nutrients in and out of cells. They regulate the balance of water, acids, and bases, and are essential in making antibodies. Proteins play a role in virtually every cellular function. For instance, proteins regulate muscle contraction and expansion and contraction of the blood vessels to maintain normal blood pressure.

The protein we eat is broken down into amino acids during digestion. These amino acids are absorbed into the bloodstream, where they travel to tissues throughout the body. Cells build up new proteins from these amino acids to serve specific functions. Generally, a lack of protein in the diet retards growth in children and causes a decrease in energy. A failure to consume adequate quantities of food energy may lead to weight loss or growth failure in children, wasting of tissues, and eventually starvation. The production of enzymes and hormones is impaired in severe protein deficiency. Young children living in poorer communities throughout the world commonly have protein-calorie malnutrition (PCM). The two clinical forms of PCM are nutritional marasmus and kwashiorkor. Marasmus is due primarily to a calorie deficiency, while kwashiorkor results from a protein deficiency. Mild or moderate PCM is much more common than these two severe forms and contributes to a slow rate of growth, poor development, increased susceptibility to infections, and eventually to the potential for permanent physical stunting.

Proteins are essential as the building blocks of our cells. It is imperative that all of us know something about them. Protein, like other nutrients, can be detrimental if it is either overconsumed or underconsumed. This nutrient, like almost everything else in our lives, must be understood and used in moderation.

How Much Protein Do We Need?

This answer is much less than you may think. Most Americans eat twice as much protein as RDAs suggest, but then again, many Americans are overweight. There are times when we may need additional amounts of protein. If we are undergoing extra physical or psychological stress or recovering from infections, we may need a protein boost. Infants, growing children, and pregnant and lactating women require the most protein per pound of ideal body weight.

To calculate specific protein needs, first calculate ideal weight by following these instructions:

Ideal body weight (allow plus or minus 10 percent for variations in body structure)

Men: 100 pounds for the first 5 feet of height, plus 6 pounds for each additional inch

Women: 100 pounds for the first 5 feet of height plus 5 pounds for each additional inch

Example: For a woman who is 5 feet, 6 inches tall, the ideal body weight is:

100 pound + (6 inches x 5 pounds/inch) = 130 pounds

To estimate her protein needs, she would use "130 pounds" as her ideal weight.

To estimate her ideal weight range, she would use the following:

130 pounds ideal weight plus or minus 10 percent

or

130 pounds plus or minus (130 divided by 10) =
130 plus/minus 13 = 117–143 pounds

Depending on the individual's body type, this estimate for ideal body weight range could be a little low. Persons with a lot of lean muscle tissue, which weighs more than fat, could weigh more than their ideal weight range and still look and feel fit and healthy. An appropriate weight is what a person feels good weighing.

Personal protein requirements can be calculated using table 5.1. Ideal weight, rather than actual weight, is used because the quantity of protein you need depends on the amount of lean tissue in the body, not body fat.

Multiply the ideal weight by the number of grams of protein needed per pound of body weight to calculate daily protein requirements.

Age Group	Protein Needs in Grams/Pound Ideal Body Weight
Babies: ages 5 months to 1 year	0.90
Children: ages 1 to 3	0.81
ages 4 to 6	0.68
ages 7 to 10	0.55
ages 11 to 14	0.45
ages 15 to 18	0.39
Adults: 19 and over	0.36
pregnant women	0.62
lactating women	0.53

TABLE 5.1 *Personal Protein Requirements*

Can Too Much Protein Be Harmful?

Over time, too much protein can contribute to the development of heart disease, osteoporosis, obesity, kidney disease, gout, and certain forms of cancer such as breast, prostate, and colon cancer.

Some of these diseases are also caused by the fact that a high protein intake is often accompanied by a high fat intake, especially in people who eat an excess of meat and milk products. In general, the average daily protein intake by adults in the United States exceeds the 0.8 to 1.6 gram per kilogram of body weight, equal to 0.36 to 0.73 grams per pound of body weight, recommended by the National Academy of Sciences. The results of one six-year study showed that women who ate beef, pork, or lamb as a main dish every day had 2.5 times the risk of developing colon cancer as women who consumed these red meats less than once a month.

Since protein is not stored in the body, stress is put on the kidneys as they try to eliminate surplus amounts. Excess protein has long been associated with the buildup of uric acid that can result in gout. If you have ever known a heavy meat eater who suffered from a throbbing big toe, you know about gout. At the same time, excess protein increases the amount of calcium excreted, creating a potential risk for osteoporosis and kidney stones. But to top it off, excess protein may make you fat. Due to the high levels of fat and cholesterol found in many animal protein-containing foods, the National Research Council, the American Heart Association, and many nurse, physician, and nutrition practitioners are recommending that smaller and fewer portions of meat and high-fat cheese be eaten.

How to Reduce Protein Intake

If you are a heavy meat eater, you may want to make a conscious effort to reduce protein intake. Begin by eliminating meat from one meal a day and using meat and poultry as a condiment rather than the entree for the second meal of the day. After a period of time, you may want to try eating meat at only one meal a day. You may want to substitute beans, lentils, tofu, and other vegetable protein sources in place of the meat and poultry. With quality meat at only one meal, you should still have sufficient intake quantities. A good rule of thumb is to limit each protein serving to 3 ounces (the size of a deck of cards) of cooked, trimmed beef, pork, lamb, poultry, or fish per meal, with a maximum of 6 ounces per day. If you want to try a meatless regime, see chapter 14 on vegetarianism.

MEAT

Meat products include beef, veal (calves), pork, lamb, and venison (deer). Meat is both caloric and fatty. Some people select marbled beef believing it to be the tastiest. The marbling, however, connotes fat, and fat is what makes meat consumption questionable as a healthy behavior.

Buying Meat

Purchase lean meats closely trimmed of fat, or trim them yourself at home. "Prime," the most heavily marbled grade of meat, has the highest fat content, followed by "Choice" and "Select." If buying veal, ask for naturally raised veal. These calves are allowed to walk and mingle in small herds. Although it remains slightly pink after cooking, naturally raised veal has the added benefit of being more flavorful and juicy than the pale white meat from calves that are formula-fed and tethered in small, cramped quarters.

Table 5.2 depicts the various nutrients in the most popular cuts of meat.

Lean Meat Cooking Tips

Keep lean meat lean. Avoid frying; instead, bake, broil, or roast on a rack. Lightly saute or stir fry with minimal oil. Marinate with spices, wine, or lemon instead of oil. For maximum tenderness, cook lean meats slowly with low or moderate moist heat. High heat toughens and dries meat. Especially avoid overcooking lean cuts, which can become dry, tough, and tasteless if cooked too long.

Storing Meat

Properly wrapped and stored, fresh steaks, chops, and roasts can be safely stored for 3 to 5 days in the refrigerator or 6 to 9 months in the freezer. Ground or stew meats and organ meats, such as heart and liver, should be used within 1 to 2 days. They may also be frozen for 3 to 4 months. Cooked meat and meat dishes can be used for leftovers for 3 to 4 days when stored in the refrigerator or 2 to 3 months in the freezer.

Beef, Pork, Lamb, & Veal	Total Calories kcal	Protein g	Carbohydrates g	Total Fat g	Saturated Fatty Acids g	Cholesterol mg	Sodium mg	Vitamin A	Vitamin C	Calcium	Iron
								% U.S. RDA			
Beef											
Top round steak	216	30	0	10	4	85	60	0	0	7	3
Sirloin steak	215	29	0	10	4	89	65	0	0	11	3
Tenderloin steak	235	27	0	13	5	85	62	0	0	7	3
Top loin steak	98	29	10	8	3	76	68	0	0	8	8
Eye of round	171	29	0	5	2	69	62	0	0	5	2
Tip round	191	28	0	8	3	81	64	0	0	5	3
Bottom round	188	29	0	7	3	78	66	0	0	5	3
Chuck arm roast	280	30	0	17	7	100	62	0	0	10	3
Ground beef, extra lean	265	28	0	16	6	99	82	0	0	9	3
Ground round	292	27	0	20	8	101	93	0	0	12	3
Pork											
Center loin chop	229	30	0	11	4	81	63	6	0	29	1
Fresh whole ham	278	27	0	18	7	94	60	10	0	7	1
Shoulder picnic cut	317	23	0	24	9	94	70	8	0	19	1
Tenderloin	201	30	0	8	3	94	64	7	1	5	1
Lamb											
Leg of lamb	258	25	0	17	7	93	66	*	*	11	2
Loin chop	316	25	0	23	10	100	77	*	*	20	2
Shoulder arm chop	278	24	0	19	8	97	78	*	*	21	2
Rib roast	359	21	0	30	13	97	73	*	*	22	2
Arm chop	281	24	0	20	8	96	77	*	*	18	2
Veal											
Cutlet (top round)	211	36	0	6	3	134	67	*	*	8	1
Sirloin	252	31	0	13	5	108	79	*	*	17	1
Ground	172	24	0	8	3	103	83	*	*	17	1

Serving Size: 3.5 oz. (trimmed to 0 fat) cooked portion broiled, braised, or roasted without additional fat, sodium, or sauces.

*indicates no available data

Data Source: USDA Agricultural Handbook

TABLE 5.2   Meat Nutrition Information

Keeping Meat Safe

The recent deaths and serious illnesses from tainted fast-food hamburgers underscore the importance of food safety. Most meat and poultry contain millions of bacteria, some of them quite dangerous. But through proper food handling, the bacteria can be prevented from multiplying to numbers large enough to cause illness. The following points should ensure safety.

1. *Cook hamburger meat thoroughly, until no pink color shows at the center of the patty.* Hamburger meat is riskier than steaks and other cuts because it is ground and mixed, giving it a much larger surface area for bacterial growth.

2. *Use a meat thermometer.* Cook all meats to an internal temperature of at least 160 degrees. Red meat is done when it is brown or gray inside. Poultry is done when its juices run clear and no pink color shows at the center or next to the bone. Rare beef does carry some bacterial risk.

3. *Wash your hands.* Wash your hands in hot, soapy water before and after handling raw meat or poultry. Wash them again during food preparation if you sneeze, cough, or blow your nose.

4. *Use separate cutting boards for preparing raw meats.* Wash cutting boards with hot, soapy water after use. Occasionally give them a second wash with a mild bleach solution and rinse with clean water.

5. *Use clean utensils.* Never use utensils that have touched raw meat and poultry without thoroughly washing them first.

6. *Use clean sponges and towels.* Clean up drippings from raw meat with a paper towel to avoid contaminating a sponge or dishcloth.

7. *Observe the "sell by" and "use by" dates.*

8. *Do not trust your nose.* Although you should not prepare meats that smell bad, do not trust your nose. You cannot smell bacteria.

9. *Never thaw meat or poultry at room temperature.* Thaw in the refrigerator or microwave oven.

10. *Do not let meat stand at room temperature for more than two hours.* Food that sits on a warming tray for a long time is especially vulnerable to bacterial growth.

11. *Store meats properly in the refrigerator.* Store raw roasts and steaks in the refrigerator no longer than 3 to 5 days, raw hamburger and stew meat no longer than 2 days, raw chicken or turkey no longer than 1 to 2 days, and leftover cooked meats no longer than 3 to 4 days.

FISH

Seafood is generally lower in calories than meat. Table 5.3 depicts the nutritional values for the 20 most commonly consumed types of seafood. Values are given for a single serving (3 oz.) of edible, cooked, skinless portion. Use this information to choose a healthy diet that includes a variety of seafood.

Selecting Fresh Fish

Whatever the variety, whole fish have certain characteristics that indicate freshness. Look for

- Bright, clear, full eyes that are often protruding. As a fish loses freshness, the eyes become cloudy, pink, and sunken.

- Firm and elastic flesh that springs back when pressed gently with the finger. With time, the flesh becomes soft and slips from the bone.

- Shiny skin with scales that adhere tightly. Characteristic colors and markings start to fade as soon as the fish leaves the water.

- A clean, pink intestinal cavity.

- A fresh, mild odor.

Fillets and fish steaks should have a firm and elastic flesh and a fresh-cut appearance with no browning or drying around the edges.

Seafood	Total Calories kcal	Protein g	Carbohydrates g	Total Fat g	Saturated Fatty Acids g	Cholesterol mg	Sodium mg	Vitamin A % U.S. RDA	Vitamin C % U.S. RDA	Calcium % U.S. RDA	Iron % U.S. RDA
Blue Crab, steamed	90	19	0	1	0	80	310	*	*	9	4
Catfish, baked	120	19	0	5	1	60	65	*	*	3	5
Clam, steamed, 12 small	130	22	4	2	0	60	95	10	*	8	130
Cod, broiled	90	19	0	1	0	50	60	*	2	*	2
Flounder, baked	100	20	0	1	0	50	85	*	*	2	2
Haddock, baked	90	20	0	1	0	60	70	*	*	4	6
Halibut, broiled	120	22	0	2	0	30	60	3	*	5	5
Lobster, broiled	100	20	1	1	0	100	320	*	*	5	2
Mackerel, Atlantic, Pacific, & Jack, broiled	190	21	0	12	3	60	95	7	*	*	9
Mahi Mahi, broiled	90	20	n/a	1	0	80	95	n/a	n/a	n/a	10
Ocean Perch, baked	100	20	0	2	0	50	80	*	*	10	6
Orange Roughy, broiled	70	16	0	1	0	20	70	*	*	*	*
Oyster, steamed, 12 medium	120	12	7	4	1	90	190	*	*	8	65
Pollack, broiled	100	21	0	1	0	80	90	*	*	*	*
Rainbow Trout, broiled	130	22	0	4	1	60	30	*	*	7	10
Rockfish, baked	100	20	0	2	0	40	65	4	*	*	3
Salmon, Atlantic/Coho, baked	150	22	0	5	0	50	50	*	2	*	4
Shark, baked	140	22	n/a	5	1	50	80	n/a	n/a	n/a	5
Scallop, broiled, 6 large or 14 small	150	29	2	1	0	60	275	*	3	2	*
Shrimp, boiled	110	22	0	2	0	160	155	*	3	3	15
Sole, broiled	100	21	0	1	0	60	90	*	*	2	2
Swordfish, broiled	130	21	0	4	1	40	110	4	*	*	5
Tuna, Yellowfin, broiled	120	25	0	1	0	50	40	n/a	n/a	n/a	4
Whiting, baked	100	19	0	1	0	70	75	2	*	5	2

Serving Size: 3 oz. cooked portion—skinless, broiled/grilled, baked, microwaved, boiled, or steamed without additional fat, sodium, or sauces.

*Contains less than 2% of U.S. RDA

Data Source: Nutritional Labeling Data provided by the Food and Drug Administration and Food Processor II™

TABLE 5.3 *Seafood Nutrition Information*

Storing Fresh Fish

Fresh fish should be kept in the coldest part of the refrigerator and cooked within 1 or 2 days.

Buying Frozen Fish

The technology of handling seafood has improved tremendously in recent years. Commercially frozen fish has been quickly frozen at its peak while still on board the fishing vessel. When properly thawed, it is comparable to fish that was never frozen and exhibits the same qualities of freshness. When buying frozen fish, look for packages that still have their original shape with the wrappings intact and no ice or blood visible.

Defrosting Frozen Fish

Place the package of frozen fish in a dish and allow it to thaw for 24 hours in the refrigerator. Fish can be thawed in its original package under cold, running water, but this method will result in a loss of flavor and texture.

Cooking Tips

Fish should be cooked according to the "ten minutes per inch" rule, based on the maximum thickness of the fish. Steaks and thicker fillets should be turned halfway through the cooking time. Pieces of fish less than 1/2-inch thick do not have to be turned. Fillets should be placed skin side down. The skin will remove easily after cooking. If fillets are rolled or stuffed, measure at the thickest point to determine cooking time. Fish is done when the flesh begins to change from translucent to opaque or white and is firm but still moist. It should flake easily with a fork.

Grilling   Place steaks or fillets on an oiled grill over medium-hot coals. Cover and cook without turning, or if left uncovered, turn halfway through cooking time. If using a stovetop grill, fill the basin with water and brush the surface of the grill lightly with oil. Cook over medium-high heat and provide adequate ventilation.

Broiling Place steaks or fillets in a broiling pan and brush with marinade. Broil 3 to 6 inches from heat, basting frequently and turning steaks halfway through cooking.

Poaching Simmer fillets or steaks in a stock, using a pan with a lid to retain heat. Turning is not necessary. Baste occasionally by spooning stock over fish.

Pan Sauteing Heat a small amount of marinade or oil in a heavy skillet. For steaks or fillets over 1/2-inch thick, turn halfway through cooking time.

Baking Preheat oven to 450°F. Bake uncovered, basting if desired.

POULTRY

Poultry is a broad classification that covers the various species of domesticated and game birds that are raised to provide food for humans. These include turkey, chicken, duck, goose, and wild birds. When cooking poultry, take the same precautions as when cooking meat or fish. Always make sure that the flesh is fully cooked before eating. If you see a pink tinge, even next to the bone, cook the poultry a little longer.

MILK AND CHEESES

The milk group includes milk, cheese, ice cream, yogurt, and kefir. The importance of milk in the diet has long been recognized. Whereas milk contains important amounts of most nutrients, it is very low in iron and ascorbic acid, and it is low in niacin. Calcium and phosphorus levels in milk are very high. Vitamin A levels are high in whole milk, but in the production of skim milk, this fat-soluble vitamin is removed. Riboflavin is present in significant quantities in milk unless the milk has been exposed to light. The composition of whole milk is approximately 4.9 percent carbohydrate, 3.5 percent fat, 3.5 percent protein, and about 87 percent water. The main carbohydrate in milk is lactose, or milk sugar. The most abundant fatty acids in milk are oleic, palmitic, and stearic acids. Milk is a complete protein food containing several protein complexes. The chief protein fraction in cow's milk is casein. The whey protein complex includes lactalbumin, lactoglobulin, and lactomucin.

Cheese is one of the oldest and most nutritious food products. It is formed by the coagulation of milk by rennet (the digestive enzyme in the stomach of the calf) or similar enzymes, and the draining off of the liquid whey. Part of the moisture is removed from the curd by cutting, warming, or pressing. Then it is usually shaped in a mold and ripened by storing for some time at a particular temperature and humidity. The ripening, or curing, process is the result of bacteriological processes. Processed cheese is a mixture of ground cheese (usually cheddar and other hard varieties), emulsifying salts such as phosphates, other ingredients such as milk powder, whey powder, and coloring and flavoring materials, and, sometimes, spices. Vegetable gum is often added to produce a chewy texture. Steam is blown into the mixture to raise the temperature to 150°F or higher, which yields a molten plasticlike mass that is then poured into a metal or ceramic container, or into portion-containers for foil wrapping.

Hard cheese, such as cheddar, is one of the most concentrated of common foods: 100 grams (about 3.5 oz.) supplies about 36 percent of the protein, 80 percent of the calcium, and 34 percent of the fat in the recommended daily allowance. Cheese is also a good source of some vitamins and minerals.

Nutritionally, milk is best preserved by condensing or drying, as none of the nutrients are lost. Conversion to cheese also is an excellent way to preserve the nutrients of milk, because virtually all the fat and most of the protein are retained, and the latter is partially digested. However, nearly all the sugar (lactose) and some of the minerals, protein, and vitamins escape into the whey. Because cheese is a high-protein food, it is an ideal nutritional replacement for meat in a vegetarian diet. It is rich in the essential amino acids, calcium, phosphorus, other minerals, and vitamins, and it has a high caloric value.

One of the primary habits you will want to develop regarding cheeses is to read the labels. Cheeses vary so greatly in fat and calorie content that you will either want to see the breakdown on the label or learn about various full cut, unlabeled products yourself. In this way, you can become a savvy cheese eater.

SUMMARY

Proteins are the most important part of nutrition. The human body is made of proteins and they play an essential role in how it functions. When dieting, when eating for energy, while exercising, during pregnancy, or in old age protein needs must be met.

6 | FATS

A generation ago we didn't know that smearing butter on sandwiches, deep fat frying, and eating red meat three times a day could be detrimental to our health. I remember my mother saving the morning bacon fat in a peanut butter jar that sat on the windowsill. It was added for flavoring to most meals and the daily fried eggs were splattered with it to cook the sunny tops. Beans were cooked with ham or bacon, and rich, full-fat butter coated everything. And, of course, the delicious country Sunday chicken was fried in lard.

These days we know a lot more and are consequently in the midst of a major dietary transition. Today, we have differentiated between "hydrogenated" and "saturated" fats and we know the difference between "polysaturated" and "monosaturated" fats. Each of these fats is different and some are better for us than others.

OVERVIEW

Lipids, which make up most of the rest of the body's weight, serve as stores of food energy in the form of fat. More complex lipids, such as phospholipids, are basic constituents of cell membranes and steroids, which include hormones that perform other vital chemical functions. The following terms describe aspects of fat that we hear about frequently, but may need to brush up on for better understanding.

Saturated Fats

Saturated fats contain large numbers of hydrogen atoms in their chemical composition. They are suspected of raising blood cholesterol levels. Most saturated fats come from animal products. *Tropical* vegetable oils (palm kernel, palm, and coconut, particularly) are the only vegetable fats that are high in saturated fats. Saturated fats have been linked to an increased risk of coronary heart disease. A higher percentage of saturated fats can increase total blood cholesterol, especially the "bad" low-density lipoproteins (LDLs). Oils and fats with a high proportion of saturated fats include palm oil, coconut oil, and lard.

Hydrogenated Fats or Trans-Fatty Acids

Hydrogenated fats have undergone a process whereby hydrogen is bubbled through a polyunsaturated fat in order to give the otherwise liquid fat a harder consistency and more stability against rancidity. An example of a hydrogenated fat is margarine. Hydrogenated fats are no more healthy than comparable animal-based saturated fats. There are also concerns as to how the chemical nature of the fat is changed during hydrogenation and how usable these hydrogenated fats are in the body.

Polyunsaturated Fats

Polyunsaturated fats are considered physiologically less threatening and tend to decrease total blood cholesterol. Unfortunately, they also lower the amount of "good" blood cholesterol, or high-density lipoproteins (HDLs). Too many polyunsaturated fats in the diet may also increase the risk of some types of cancer. Linoleic acid (a polyunsaturated fat) has been found to enhance the growth of breast, pancreatic, and possibly colon cancer in rats (Carter, 1985). Oils and fats with a high proportion of polyunsaturated fats include soybean oil, corn oil, sunflower oil, safflower oil, and cottonseed oil. Vegetable oils (corn, cottonseed, soybean, safflower) contain large percentages of the polyunsaturated fatty acid linolenic acid. Peanut and sesame oils are fairly high in linolenic acid.

Monounsaturated Fats

Monounsaturated fats seem to help reduce levels of LDLs while preserving the beneficial HDLs. Oils high in monounsaturated fats include canola oil, olive oil, high-oleic safflower oil, peanut oil, and sesame oil. Studies show that in cultures where people use olive oil as the predominant fat, there tends to be a lower incidence of heart disease. An added advantage of monounsaturated fats is their naturally high resistance to rancidity. Since monounsaturated fats are basically healthy, and we do need fats in our diets, some facts about olive oil follow.

Olive Oil   Olive oil is one of the few oils in the world pressed from a fruit. It has been savored by Greeks and Southern Italians for centuries, and these populations have surprisingly low rates of cardiovascular disease even with fairly high consumption of this fat. Olive oil is available in the following types:

> *Extra-virgin*—the top grade, most expensive of the oils; naturally contains less than 1 percent acid. It is the most flavorful, with a fruity or peppery olive taste.
>
> *Virgin*—contains 1 percent to 3.3 percent acid.
>
> *Refined*—the lowest and least expensive grade; contains more than 3.3 percent acid.
>
> *Pure*—a blend of virgin or extra-virgin with refined olive oil; contains no more than 3.3 percent acid.

Some information on the background of olive oils: where they grow, how they are harvested, and so on, follows.

- *Geographic and seasonal facts.* Soil, climate, and particular weather conditions all affect the characteristics of agricultural products such as grapes, milk, and olives. That is why only specific regions of the world, such as the Middle East and Mediterranean countries, cultivate olive trees.

- *Time of harvest.* The flavor of olives differs greatly from one plant to another. Flavor is due partly to the ripeness of the olive. Green olives picked in September or October have a sharper, fruitier flavor and a greener color than the darker, riper olives picked in November and December, which are sweeter and more subtle.

- *Method of harvest.* The best olive oils are made from hand-picked olives. Hand-picked olives do not get bruised and can be selected for the desired ripeness. These olives are made into the virgin or extra-virgin oils. Lower-quality oils are made from olives that have been mechanically harvested or have fallen to the ground.

- *Olive oil production.* The very best oils are from olives that are "cold-pressed" between mill stones after drying for 2 to 3 days to reduce the water content. Traditional small olive oil producers run their mills continuously so the olives can be pressed at their peak condition.

- *Care of olive oil.* Store olive oil in a cool, dark place, making sure it is not exposed to direct light. In hot climates, it can be stored in the refrigerator, but unrefined extra-virgin oil will solidify. It will melt back into a liquid upon standing at room temperature. It is best to use a bottle or tin of olive oil within a year of purchase.

- *Uses for olive oil.* Olive oil is excellent when combined with vinegar for salad dressings, tossed with pasta, used as a saute base for stovetop meals, or substituted for butter or margarine on bread.

- *Caloric content.* Like all oils, olive oil contains 120 calories and 14 grams of fat per tablespoon. Consequently, no matter how good a replacement it is for other kinds of fat, it should be used with discretion.

CHOLESTEROL

Cholesterol is a waxy substance made primarily in the liver and in the cells lining the small intestine. It is an essential constituent of cell membranes and nerve fibers, and is a building block of certain hormones. It is found in all body tissues, but the cholesterol that circulates in the blood creates the most concern. Fats (triglycerides) and cholesterol are transported through the bloodstream in protein-wrapped clusters called lipoproteins, which are assembled in the liver and intestinal tract. These lipoproteins are labeled according to their "density," based on the proportion of triglycerides, phospholipids, cholesterol, and protein they contain.

Total Cholesterol

Total cholesterol reflects the total amount of artery-clogging cholesterol in the blood. The National Cholesterol Education Program designates blood levels less than 200 mg/dl as desirable; levels between 200 and 240 mg/dl as borderline-high; and those over 240 mg/dl as indicative of a greater risk of heart disease. The three other lipid values are measurements of lipoproteins, the special proteins that carry cholesterol through the vascular system.

Very Low Density Lipoproteins (VLDL)   VLDLs contain 55 to 65 percent triglycerides, 5 to 10 percent protein, 10 to 15 percent cholesterol, and 15 to 20 percent phospholipids. Their job is to carry triglycerides to the cells for use or to other parts of the body for storage. After the VLDLs deposit their triglycerides and undergo other changes, they become low density lipoproteins.

Low Density Lipoproteins (LDL)   LDLs contain 45 percent cholesterol, 25 percent moderate protein, 10 percent triglycerides, and 22 percent phospholipids. These lipoproteins have become known as *bad* cholesterol because after they deliver the cholesterol actually needed by the cells, they deposit any excess in arterial walls and other tissues.

High Density Lipoproteins (HDL)   HDLs contain the highest amount of protein (45 to 50 percent), 5 percent triglycerides, 20 percent cholesterol, and 30 percent phospholipids. HDL lipoproteins pick up the cholesterol deposits and bring them to the liver for recycling or disposal; thus they are known as the *good* cholesterol. A higher proportion of HDL lipoproteins to LDL lipoproteins represents more active cholesterol, a lowered risk of developing atherosclerosis, and a lower risk of heart attack and stroke.

Sensitivity to Dietary Cholesterol

It is theorized that 20 to 30 percent of the population are genetically hypersensitive to dietary cholesterol and, therefore, have blood cholesterol levels that increase when they eat high-cholesterol foods. Since there is no simple test for cholesterol hypersensitivity, it is suggested that everyone monitor their intake of dietary cholesterol.

Cholesterol is found only in foods of animal origin: meat, eggs, poultry, fish, and dairy products, including butter. Fruits, vegetables, grains, and legumes contain no cholesterol. Saturated fats in foods usually stimulate the production of LDL (bad) cholesterol and raise overall cholesterol levels. Therefore, even if a low-cholesterol diet is maintained, a diet high in saturated fats can still mean trouble.

New understanding of the important role of HDLs in protecting against heart disease led a National Institutes of Health panel to recommend that all adults know their HDL and total cholesterol levels. Bringing abnormal lipid levels within normal parameters lowers the risk factors for heart disease. For every 1 percent drop in total cholesterol, the risk of heart disease declines 2 to 3 percent. And every 1 mg/dl higher increment in HDL reduces heart disease by another 2 to 3 percent.

Taking cholesterol-lowering drugs can reduce levels. A low-fat diet lowers cholesterol about 10 percent, whereas adding cholesterol-lowering drugs to a low-fat diet can bring a 20 percent reduction. The decision to supplement a low-fat diet with pharmaceutical aids depends on an individual's complete risk profile: total cholesterol and lipoprotein levels, family history, prior myocardial infarction or stroke, smoking, obesity, and hypertension.

RISK FACTORS

Risk factors are based on determination of high, moderate, or low risk for heart disease. Risk factors are determined by evaluating the person's current cholesterol level, weight, prior family history, smoking history, exercise patterns, and intake of high cholesterol and highly saturated foods. The following recommendations of the American Heart Association are based on risk group category.

High. Eat no more than 20 percent of your total calories from fat, and reduce cholesterol to 100–150 mg per day.

Moderate. Eat no more than 25 percent of your total calories from fat, and reduce cholesterol to 200–250 mg per day.

Low. Eat no more than 30 percent of your total calories from fat, and reduce cholesterol to 200–300 mg per day.

Fats are usually calculated or measured in grams of fat. Table 6.1 lists the number of grams of fat for most of the common foods. The following list explains ways to reduce fat consumption.

1. Know your numbers. Total cholesterol should be less than 200 mg/dl. Levels over 240 mg/dl demand attention. HDL cholesterol should be over 35 mg/dl. Less than 35 mg/dl demands attention. Above 45 mg/dl is even better. LDL cholesterol should be less than 160 mg/dl. The ratio of total cholesterol to HDL cholesterol is best if below 4.5; above 5.5 is undesirable. Lipoprotein should be less than 0.3 g/l.

2. Get a lipid analysis. Do not rely on a simple cholesterol test. Findings indicate abnormal levels of lipids can be corrected when we know our levels and are motivated to change.

3. Follow dietary restrictions prior to the test. A 12-hour fast is necessary for an accurate measurement of LDL cholesterol and triglycerides.

4. If the results are normal, have a follow-up lipid test every five years. If one or more values fall outside the desirable range, get more frequent tests.

5. Make necessary lifestyle changes. A low-fat, low-cholesterol diet will help bring lipid abnormalities in line. Maintaining optimum weight and regular exercise can boost HDL levels.

6. Eliminate other risk factors. If you smoke, stop. If you are overweight, reduce. If you are sedentary, begin to move. Seek medical attention for diabetes, hypertension, or when there is a family history of dietary related problems.

TABLE 6.1 Grams of Fat for Common Foods

Meats—Poultry (1 oz. cooked)	Grams
Chicken, broilers or fryers, dark meat with skin, roasted	4
Chicken, dark meat without skin, roasted	3
Chicken, light meat with skin, roasted	3
Chicken, light meat without skin, roasted	1
Chicken frankfurter, about 2	6
Turkey bacon	10
Turkey bologna, about 3½ slices	4
Turkey frankfurter, about 2	5
Turkey, light meat with skin, roasted	5
Turkey, light meat without skin, roasted	1

Meats—Beef (1 oz. cooked)	Grams
Bologna, cured, 3–4 slices	8
Chuck, arm pot roast, lean only, braised	3
Frankfurter, cured, about 2	8
Ground, lean, broiled	5
Hot Dog, 97% fat free	0.5
Hot Dog, cured, 90% fat free	3
Round, bottom round, lean only, braised	3
Round, top round, lean only, broiled	2
Sausage, cured, cooked, about 2	8

Meats—Pork (1 oz. cooked)	Grams
Bacon, Canadian	1
Breakfast Strips	7
Bacon, fried	14
Cured ham, boneless, regular, roasted	3
Cured, smoked link sausage, grilled	9
Fresh, loin, center loin, lean and fat, roasted	6
Fresh, loin, tenderloin, lean only, roasted	1

Meats—Fish and Shellfish (1 oz. cooked)	Grams
Haddock, dry heat	0.3
Salmon, sockeye, dry heat	3
Tuna, bluefin, dry heat	2
Lobster, northern	0.2
Oyster, Eastern, moist heat	1
Shrimp, mixed species	0.3

Dairy and Egg Products	Grams
American processed cheese food, 1 oz.	7
Cheddar, 1 oz.	9
Cottage cheese, creamed, 4 oz.	5
Cottage cheese, 1% fat, 4 oz.	1
Cream cheese, 1 oz.	10
Mozzarella, 1 oz.	6
Mozzarella, part skim, 1 oz.	5
Muenster, 1 oz.	9
Parmesan, 1 oz.	9
Provolone, 1 oz.	8
Ricotta, part skim, 4 oz.	9
Ricotta, whole milk, 4 oz.	15
Swiss, 1 oz.	8

Eggs	Grams
Egg, chicken, white	tr
Egg, chicken, whole	6

Frozen Desserts	Grams
Frozen yogurt, fruit-flavored, low-fat	2
Fudgesicle	0.2
Frozen yogurt, nonfat	0
Frozen yogurt, regular	7
Ice cream, vanilla, regular	14
Ice milk, vanilla, soft serve	5
Pudding pops, 1 pop	3
Sherbet, orange	4

Milk (8 oz.)	Grams
Buttermilk	2
Chocolate shake	11
Low-fat milk, 1% fat	3
Low-fat milk, 2% fat	5
Skim milk	0.4
Whole milk, 3.3% fat	8

Yogurt (4 oz.)	Grams
Plain yogurt	4
Plain yogurt, low-fat	0.2

Nuts and Seeds (1 oz.)	Grams		Grams
Almonds	15	Trail mix	12
Cashew nuts	13	Sunflower seeds	14
Peanuts	14	Walnuts	18
Pecans	18		

Breads, Cereals, Pasta, Rice, and Dried Peas and Beans

	Grams		Grams
Biscuits, buttermilk or oven-ready, 3"	3	Rolls, brown & serve, 1 each	2
Croissant, 4½"	12	Rolls, crescent, 1 each	4–6
Doughnut, 3/4"	12	Rolls, dinner, butterflake, 1 each	5
Danish	8	Waffle, 7"	13
French, 1–2 oz.	1	Waffle, lite	2
Muffin, 2½"	5–6	Wheat/white bread, 2 slices	1
Pancake, 4"	2	Turnover, cherry	19
Raisin, biscuit	7	Granola type (¼ cup)	6

Pasta (1 cup)

	Grams		Grams
Chow mein noodles	11	Egg noodles, cooked	2

Sweets and Snacks

Cakes and Pies

	Grams		Grams
Apple pie, ⅛ of 9" pie	13	Lemon meringue pie, ⅛ of 9" pie	
Cream pie, ⅛ of 9" pie	17		11
Gingerbread, ⅛ of 8" cake	4	Pound cake, 1/17 of loaf	5
Layer cake with icing, ⅛ of 9" cake	8–9	Pudding, ½ cup	4

Candy

	Grams		Grams
Banana chips, ¼ cup	6	Chocolate chips, ¼ cup	12
Butterfingers/Nestle Crunch, ¼ cup	7	Fudge, 1 oz.	3
		Gummi Bears, ¼ cup	0
		Jelly beans, ¼ cup	0

Sweets and Snacks (cont.)	Grams		Grams
Candy			
M&M (peanut), ¼ cup	14	Raisinettes, ¼ cup	8
M&M (plain), 1 oz.	9	Reese's Pieces, ¼ cup	10
Milk chocolate, plain, ¼ cup	13	Yogurt-covered raisins, ¼ cup	16
Snacks			
Corn chips, 1 oz.	9	Potato chips, 1 oz.	10
Popcorn, with oil, 1 cup	3	Pretzels, stick, 2¼", 10 pretzels	tr
Popcorn, air popped, 1 cup	tr		
Miscellaneous			
Pizza, cheese ⅛ of 15" diameter	9		
Fats and Oils			
Margarine, diet, 1 tsp	2	Margarine, soft, tub, 1 tsp.	2
Margarine, liquid, bottled, 1 tsp.	3	Margarine, stick, 1 tsp.	4
Salad Dressing (1 Tbsp.)			
Bleu cheese	8	Low calorie	1–2
French	6	Mayonnaise	11
Imitation mayonnaise	3	Ranch	6
Italian	7	Thousand Island	6
Other			
Avocado, Florida	27	Olives, green, 4 medium	1.5
Gravies, canned, ½ cup	3–7	Peanut butter, 1 tbsp.	7
Nondairy creamer, powdered, 1 tsp.	1	Sour cream, 2 tbsp.	5

TABLE 6.1 Grams of Fat for Common Foods (continued)

HOW MUCH FAT DO WE NEED?

Most nutritionists concur that we need to limit all fats to 30 percent of our total caloric intake. Of that amount, saturated fats should constitute less than 10 percent of our total daily requirements. The remaining 20 percent should be divided between polyunsaturated and monounsaturated fats. This means that on a diet of approximately 2,000 calories per day, 600 of the calories may come from fats. The American Heart Association recommends more specific guidelines and suggests that fewer than 10 percent of daily calories come from saturated fats and fewer than 10 percent come from polyunsaturated fats. Monounsaturated fats should make up the rest. Since a tablespoon of oil contains about 120 calories, we can consume up to 5 tablespoons of oil and still remain within the 30 percent guideline if our calorie needs are around 2,000 calories per day. However, these 5 tablespoons also include all the hidden fats found in baked goods, candy, meats, fish, poultry, nuts, seeds, peanut butter, eggs, and salad dressings, as well as the oil and butter we use to saute or flavor foods. If we take in 2,000 calories a day, that means consuming fewer than 67 grams of fat (1 gram of fat provides 9 calories, so 67 grams x 9 calories/gram = 603 calories). If we consume 1,500 calories a day we need to keep daily fat intake under 50 grams.

What Is the Difference Between Margarine and Butter?

Butter   Butter is a delicately flavored dairy food made from milk fat to which salt and coloring are usually added. It is believed that the saturated fatty acids found in butter, milk, and other animal products can raise the level of cholesterol in the blood, thus leading to arteriosclerosis.

Margarine   Margarine is a hydrogenated fat similar to the hardened vegetable shortenings sold in cans. The hydrogenation process involves adding hydrogen atoms to soybean, corn, and other liquid oils to make the oils more solid and resistant to rancidity. This process changes many of the unsaturated fatty acids, making them more saturated and transforming their chemical structures. Appropriately, these altered fats are called "trans-fatty acids." The more solid the margarine, the more trans-fatty acids it contains. Consequently, stick margarines contain more trans-fatty acids than tub brands, and tubs have more than the squeeze-bottle products. Concerns are that trans-fatty acids may increase the risk of heart disease, cancer, and possibly other problems. Margarine has been found to contain transmonounsaturated fatty acids which form during the processing. These fatty acids raise cholesterol levels.

Recent reports cite that diets high in trans-fatty acids raise the bad LDL cholesterol almost as much as saturated fats. More significant is that, unlike the other diets, the trans-fatty diet also lowers the good HDL cholesterol, suggesting that it may increase coronary risk as much as the high saturated-fat diet.

Since margarine and butter both can cause problems, choosing one over the other can be difficult. Minimizing both and alternating which one you use could be a way of improving your odds. For other ideas, read on.

ALTERNATIVES TO BUTTER OR MARGARINE

If both butter and margarine are dubious for good health, then what can we use for flavoring and cooking? Probably the best place to start is to reduce all fats in general and minimize foods high in saturated fats. If you choose to use margarine, try liquid or "squeeze" margarines instead of the more hydrogenated stick versions. The first ingredient listed on the label should be a liquid rather than a partially hydrogenated oil and the product should contain twice as much unsaturated fat as saturated. Avoid any brands with preservatives and artificial color.

The best alternative may be to substitute natural monounsaturated oils. Liquid vegetable oils (olive, canola, or peanut) can be used in cooking and baking. Bite-size pieces of fresh breads can be dipped into a small saucer of olive oil.

BASIC CHANGES

The easiest way to maintain a low-fat, low-cholesterol meal plan is to use low-fat products and to prepare foods with minimal fat additives. Begin your dietary lifestyle change by choosing one, two, or three of the following changes and gradually include the others.

- Broil, bake, or steam instead of frying foods in fat.
- Use skim milk or low-fat milk and milk products.
- Limit intake of meats, fish, and poultry to 5 to 6 ounces per day and trim the fat.
- Substitute meatless or "low-meat" main dishes for regular entrees (see chapter 14 on vegetarianism).
- Limit use of shrimp, lobster, sardines, and organ meats.
- Eat fatty fish once or twice weekly. They contain Omega-3 fatty acids, which lower blood cholesterol and triglycerides.
- Avoid foods containing hydrogenated vegetable shortenings, lard, hydrogenated or partially hydrogenated vegetable oils, coconut oil, palm kernel oil, and palm oil.
- Use vegetable oils in cooking. Use no more than a total of 5 to 8 teaspoons of fats and oils per day for cooking, baking, and salads.
- Use no more than 3 egg yolks per week.

Try using egg whites or cholesterol-free frozen egg products in cooking or baking. In baking, 1 whole egg equals 2 egg whites plus 1 teaspoon of oil. Many recipes work with 2 egg whites substituted for 1 whole egg.

RESEARCH STUDIES

In a study reported in the Journal of the National Cancer Institute researchers took dietary histories from 240 patients undergoing treatment for stage I or stage II breast cancer and followed their progress for four years. They found that among women with estrogen-responsive tumors, low dietary fat intake was linked to treatment success. Women who experienced a recurrence reported higher intakes of total fat, saturated fat, and polyunsaturated fat than did the successfully treated women. When examining the women's percentages of daily calories derived from fat, researchers found that for every 1 percent increase in fat, the risk of recurrence increased 10 percent ("Breast cancer recurrence," 1993).

We know that regular aerobic exercise raises HDL, the good cholesterol, and lowers triglycerides. One study suggests that strength training may have other positive effects by lowering both total cholesterol and LDL (bad) cholesterol levels in premenopausal women. In a recent study, two groups of women were assigned to either an experimental exercise group or a no-exercise control group. All participants continued their usual eating patterns. Those in the experimental group engaged in a supervised strength training program for one hour, 3 times a week. At the end of 5 months, the exercise experimental group showed significant declines in cholesterol levels, lowering their total cholesterol by an average of 13 points and their LDL cholesterol by an average of 14 points ("Weight training lowers," 1993).

SUMMARY

Fats play a very complex part in our lives. Having too much or too little of this lipid can affect our health. In this aspect of our nutrition, the best objective to seek is moderation.

References

Carter, C. A. (1985). Requirement of essential fatty acid for mammary tumorigenesis in the rat. *Cancer Research, 45*, 1997–2001.

Pariza, M. W. (1988). Dietary fat and cancer: Evidence and research needs. *Annals Review Nutrition, 8*, 167–183.

Staff. Breast cancer recurrence linked to fat. (1993). *University of Texas Lifetime Health Letter,* 5(3): 8.

Staff. Weight training lowers women's cholesterol. (1993). *University of Texas Lifetime Health Letter,* 5(4): 8.

7 CARBOHYDRATES

Susie was cute. The only problem was that she was round, entirely too round for what she should be in her late twenties. True, she had two children, but it had been four years since the last baby was born. Despite how she tried, the pounds and flab prevailed. Susie, like many women, remained chubby after childbirth. She was embarrassed by her weight and wore large, loose-fitting clothes. She opted to wear scrubs and work in an out-of-the-way area in the hospital. She felt comfortable there, especially since most of her nurse colleagues were plump too. How did Susie get this way? In this chapter, we will explore the world of carbohydrates and their role in healing nutrition. We will attempt to answer the question about Susie's weight. Carbohydrates are essential for good health, but like all other foods, they must be consumed in moderation.

OVERVIEW

Carbohydrates are the most abundant and least expensive food sources of energy. Important dietary carbohydrates are divided into two basic groups: starches and sugars. Starches, which may be converted into utilizable sugars in plants or in the human body, are supplied in grains, pulses, tubers, and some rhizomes and roots. Sugars occur in many plants and fruits. The most important food commodity among the sugars is sucrose, which is obtained from sugarcane or the sugar beet.

Carbohydrates, which include cellulose, starches, sugars, and many other compounds, are the most abundant single class of organic substances found in nature. They are formed in green plants and certain bacteria by photosynthesis, in which energy derived from sunlight is used for the assimilation of carbon dioxide from the air. If carbon dioxide, water, minerals, and an appropriate inorganic source of nitrogen are available, these organisms, with the aid of solar energy, can synthesize all the different carbohydrates, proteins, and lipids they need for their existence. Other organisms cannot do this. It follows that life on Earth ultimately depends upon this process of carbon dioxide assimilation in which carbohydrates are the first intermediates.

In animal tissues, acid carbohydrates occur in the cell coats of cartilage, bone, and other tissues and form the ground substance between connective tissue cells. The cell walls of bacteria consist of a rigid framework of sugar-polymer chains linked to peptide chains. The glycoproteins, which contain covalently attached carbohydrate groups, are widely distributed in cell membranes. In red blood corpuscles, the carbohydrate side chains determine the blood group type.

Carbohydrates also serve as storage products of energy. The principal storage forms are starch in plants and glycogen in animal tissues. Glycogen consists of polymers, or chains of glucose, that are deposited in cells in the form of granules when a surplus of glucose is available. In times of metabolic need, the polymers are broken down by enzymatic action and become fuel.

Single units of carbohydrates known as monosaccharides, or simple sugars, are compounds with either an aldehyde group or a ketone group. Monosaccharides are classified as trioses, tetroses, pentoses, and so on, indicating the number of carbon atoms in a molecule.

The use of carbohydrates by oxidation occurs in a reaction that is the reverse of that of photosynthesis. In plants, glucose is stored as starch and sucrose. In humans, excess glucose is stored as glycogen and is also converted to fat and stored in adipose tissues. Carbohydrate metabolic processes such as these are subject to regulatory controls in which various hormones play a predominant role.

SUGAR

Carbohydrates include simple sugars and giant polymers of such sugars. Sugars serve as sources of cellular energy, as building blocks for certain complex molecules, and as a way to store energy in the form of glycogen. Sugars are a diverse and important subdivision of naturally occurring carbohydrates. They are generally sweet tasting, dissolve easily in water, and form white or clear crystals when purified. Common table sugar, or sucrose, is but one of many kinds of sugars. Sugars are rapidly digested and provide a quick source of energy. They play an important but often controversial role in the diet.

Types of Sugars

1. Simple sugars, or monosaccharides, have 3 to 7 carbon atoms, in either a chain or a ring structure. Glucose and fructose are representative monosaccharides. Glucose is the sugar into which all digested carbohydrates are metabolized in the body. The term *blood sugar* refers to glucose levels in the blood. A malfunctioning of glucose metabolism can result in hypoglycemia, or high blood sugar. Glucose is used commercially as a sweetener, especially in wines and drugs. Fructose is used both as a sweetener and as a food preservative. The simple sugars ribose and deoxyribose are major constituents of the nucleic acids RNA and DNA, respectively.

2. Disaccharides consist of two simple sugars linked together. Maltose, for instance, is composed of two glucose molecules, and lactose consists of a glucose and a galactose molecule. Sucrose can be broken down into the simple sugars glucose and fructose. Large chains of simple sugars form such polysaccharides as cellulose, glycogen, and starch.

3. Sugarcane and sugar beets are the principal commercial sources of sucrose. Maple sap, sorghum, and some palm and date trees also yield limited quantities of sucrose.

FRUITS AND VEGETABLES

Remember when you were a child? If you lived on a farm or in a family who grew gardens, summertime may remind you of the abundance of fresh fruits and vegetables. Plates heaped with fresh green beans and new red potatoes were common fare. Desserts were berry pies or cobblers and Sunday afternoons always included vine-ripened watermelons. Ripe, dripping, succulent tomatoes were available directly from the vine. The freshest of healthy fruits and vegetables were a part of everyday summer life. With careful shopping they still can be today.

Vegetables

Most vegetables are important sources of minerals, vitamins, and cellulose. Some vegetables, such as potatoes, corn, and peas, contribute appreciable quantities of starch and, in some people, may be the culprit in excess calorie intake. A 1/2-cup serving of these vegetables, which have visible, white starch in the center, is equivalent in calories to one slice of bread. Balancing your intake of starchy vegetables with plenty of low-calorie vitamin- and mineral-rich ones, such as carrots, broccoli, and spinach is vital to a healthy diet.

Vegetables, particularly spinach, beans, and soybean products, contain large amounts of the minerals calcium and iron. Greens are high in calcium, while lentils and split peas are high in iron. Vegetables also help to meet the body's need for sodium, chloride, cobalt, copper, magnesium, manganese, phosphorus, and potassium. Carotenes (the precursor of vitamin A) and ascorbic acid (vitamin C) are abundant in many vegetables. Vegetables are useful in the diet for their cellulose content. Very little, if any, cellulose is digested in the body, but cellulose provides the roughage required to promote motility of food through the intestines.

Fruits

One of the best things about fresh fruit is that it is filling without adding too many calories. For the same number of calories as a regular-sized candy bar, you could eat 3 apples, which contain virtually no fat. Citrus fruits are a valuable source of vitamin C, and yellow fruits, such as peaches, contain carotene. Dried fruits contain an ample amount of iron, although these fruits contain more calories in a smaller volume. Figs and oranges are excellent sources of calcium.

Like vegetables, fruits have a high cellulose content and provide fiber to protect against hemorrhoids, diverticulitis, and some forms of colon cancer. The fruit fiber pectin seems to lower blood cholesterol levels and evidence suggests that this fiber may help regulate blood pressure. Many fruits are rich in potassium, which is necessary for muscle contraction, maintenance of fluid and electrolyte balance in cells, transmission of nerve impulses, and energy release during metabolism.

To get the most nutritional value from fruit, buy it as ripe as possible and eat it within a few days. The nutrients begin to diminish after the fruits are picked. Table 7.1 depicts the nutritional benefits of the most popular fruits.

FRUITS	BENEFITS
Apple	A good source of fiber
Apricot	Rich in beta-carotene; also contains potassium; a good source of fiber
Banana	High in potassium and vitamin B-6; a good source of fiber
Blackberry	Contains vitamin C; a good source of fiber
Cantaloupe	Rich in beta-carotene, vitamin C, thiamine, and potassium
Cherry	Contains potassium
Grapefruit	High in vitamin C
Grape	High in fiber
Honeydew Melon	High in vitamin C, thiamine, and potassium
Kiwi Fruit	Especially rich in vitamin C; good source of fiber
Mango	High in beta-carotene and vitamin C; good source of fiber
Nectarine	High in beta-carotene; contains vitamin E and potassium; good source of fiber
Orange	Especially rich in vitamin C; a good source of fiber
Papaya	High in vitamin C; also contains beta-carotene and potassium
Peach	High in beta-carotene; a good source of fiber
Pear	A good source of fiber; also contains potassium
Pineapple	High in potassium; contains vitamin C
Plum	A good source of vitamin A and fiber
Raspberry	High in niacin; also contains vitamin C; a good source of fiber
Strawberry	Especially rich in vitamin C; a good source of fiber
Watermelon	Rich in beta-carotene and potassium; contains vitamins B-6, C, and thiamine

TABLE 7.1 *Nutritional Benefits of Fresh Fruits*

Table 7.2 details nutrient information of the most available fruits.

GRAINS

Cereal grains are the least expensive source of calories for human consumption. An important energy source, they supply most of the carbohydrates in the human diet throughout the world. The proteins, lipids, vitamins, and minerals contained in cereals are also of considerable nutritional importance. The carbohydrate content of cereals ranges from 60 to 80 percent; lipid content ranges from 2 to 7 percent. The variability of the constituents is illustrated by the range of protein content within the grains: barley, 8 to 21 percent; corn, 8 to 17 percent; rye, 8 to 10 percent; wheat, 8 to 22 percent. The extent and method of processing drastically alter the vitamin, mineral, and lipid values.

Most grains are milled to separate the floury endosperm from the bran and germ, which can cause rancidity. The germ is nutritious, however, and is often added to food products after being dried and rolled. The oil extracted from the germ is refined for salad or cooking use. Most processed by-products of grain are used as feed. Flour is used in various types of baked and cereal products, pasta products, and gravies. Pearled, rolled, flaked, ground, and cut grains are used in breakfast foods, soup, meal, hominy, and specialty items.

RESEARCH ON CHOLESTEROL

In a study about reducing cholesterol levels, 621 men at risk of developing heart disease were divided into 2 groups. For 4 weeks, both groups followed the prudent diet recommended by the American Heart Association, with less than 30 percent of calories derived from fat and fewer than 300 milligrams of dietary cholesterol per day. At the end of 4 weeks, one group added more fruits and vegetables to their diet, while the control group continued on the prudent diet. The results of the study showed that the total cholesterol in the experimental group eating more

Fruit	Total Calories kcal	Protein g	Carbohydrates g	Total Fat g	Dietary Fiber mg	Sodium mg	Vitamin A % U.S. RDA	Vitamin C	Calcium	Iron
Apple, 1 med.	80	0	18	1	5	0	*	6	*	*
Apricot, 2 med.	35	1	8	0	1	1	18	12	*	2
Avocado, 1/3 med.	120	1	2	12	2	5	*	5	*	*
Banana, 1 med.	120	1	28	1	3	0	*	15	*	*
Blackberry, 1 cup	75	1	18	1	10	0	2	50	5	5
Blueberry, 1 cup	80	1	21	1	4	9	*	32	*	2
Cantaloupe, 1 cup cubed	45	1	11	0	1	12	43	93	2	2
Carambala (starfruit), 1 med.	40	1	10	0	2	3	6	50	*	2
Casaba melon, 1 cup cubed	45	1	11	0	2	20	*	45	*	4
Cherry, 1 cup	90	1	19	1	3	0	*	10	2	*
Coconut, 1"×1.5" piece	80	1	3	8	2	5	*	2	*	3
Cranberry, 1 cup	50	0	12	0	4	1	*	15	*	*
Figs, 2 med.	75	1	19	0	4	7	*	3	4	2
Grapes, 1.5 cups	85	1	24	0	2	3	3	9	2	2
Grapefruit, 1/2 med.	50	1	14	0	6	0	6	90	4	*
Honeydew melon, 1 cup cubed	60	1	16	0	2	17	*	70	*	*
Kiwi, 2 med.	90	1	18	1	4	0	2	230	4	4
Kumquat, 6 med.	70	1	19	0	4	7	3	72	5	2
Loquat, 10 med.	50	0	12	0	0	1	15	2	*	2
Lemon, 1 med.	18	0	4	0	0	10	*	35	2	*
Lime, 1 med.	20	0	7	0	3	1	*	35	2	2
Mango, 1/2 med.	65	1	18	0	4	2	40	48	*	*
Nectarine, 1 med.	70	1	16	1	3	0	20	10	*	*
Orange, 1 med.	50	1	13	0	6	0	*	120	4	*
Papaya, 1/2 med.	60	1	15	0	3	5	4	27	*	5
Passion fruit, 3 small	55	1	13	0	9	15	4	27	*	5
Peach, 2 med.	70	1	19	0	1	0	20	20	*	*
Pear, 1 med.	100	1	25	1	4	1	*	10	2	2
Persimmon, 1/2 large	60	0	16	0	2	1	18	10	*	*
Pineapple, 1/2" slice	90	1	21	1	2	10	*	35	*	*
Plantain, 1/2 med	80	1	21	0	3	3	7	20	*	2
Plum, 2 med.	70	1	17	1	1	0	9	20	*	*
Pomegranate, 1/2 med.	50	1	13	0	1	2	*	8	*	*
Prickly pear, 1 med.	40	1	10	1	2	5	*	23	6	2
Raspberry, 1 cup	60	1	14	1	8	0	*	52	2	4
Strawberry, 8 med.	50	1	13	0	30	0	*	140	2	2
Tamarind, 1 med.	5	0	1	0	0	1	*	*	*	*
Tangerine, 2 med.	70	1	19	0	2	2	30	85	2	*
Watermelon, 2 cups cubed	80	1	19	0	1	10	8	25	*	2

*less than 2%

Data Source: Nutritional Labeling Data provided by the Food and Drug Administration and Food Processor II™

TABLE 7.2   Fruit Nutrition Information

fruits and vegetables dropped 6.5 percent and LDL (bad) cholesterol dropped 7.3 percent, compared with no change in the control group. In addition, the experimental group showed improvements in HDL (good) cholesterol, triglyceride levels, and blood glucose levels. The researchers speculated that the positive effects might be attributed to the soluble fiber and/or antioxidants found in fruits and vegetables ("Fruits and vegetables," 1992).

CARBOHYDRATE ADDICTION

Not all of us can eat carbohydrates with impunity. Some of us get a taste and then develop a craving. Some nutritionists believe that this craving is a carbohydrate addiction characterized by a compelling desire for high-carbohydrate foods such as candy, ice cream, pastries, cookies, sugary sodas, cakes, and pies. This disorder, known as hyperinsulinemia, strikes a lot of us, causing us to gain large amounts of weight due to the cravings and subsequent high-volume intake. It is hypothesized that it is a hormonal imbalance due to overproduction of insulin in the body.

It is now thought that insulin levels in our systems affect food cravings. In experiments, volunteers were hooked up to IVs through which insulin and glucose were added to their blood. In the placebo group, nothing changed. Throughout the procedure, their level of hunger did not increase. In the control group, however, the higher the amount of insulin that was added to the blood, the hungrier the person felt, and the more cravings they mentioned.

Now there are ways to keep this "disorder" under control. One way is to eat a nutritious diet while limiting the number of carbohydrates. To achieve balance, three meals per day or several smaller nutritious snacks per day are essential. Another regulator of insulin is an odd little trace mineral called chromium. This mineral is thought to be deficient in most of the population because it is lost in food processing. Regular exercise also seems to be important in stopping hyperinsulinemia because it seems to increase the number of insulin receptors in muscle cells, getting insulin out of the bloodstream. Without exercise, insulin remains in the bloodstream and can cause excessive hunger and other unpleasant symptoms.

To avoid food cravings, eat three sensible meals per day, get enough vitamins and minerals, control intake of high-carbohydrate foods, and exercise regularly. For the other basic components of a nutritious diet, refer to chapters 5 and 6.

SUMMARY

Carbohydrates give us energy and endurance. Carbohydrates are something that many of us eat too much of, but when we learn how to moderate our intake, they can become the mainstay of our diets.

Reference

Staff. Fruits and vegetables lower cholesterol. (1992). *University of Texas Lifetime Health Letter,* 4 (12), 6.

8 VITAMINS AND MINERALS

Do you or your clients need vitamin and mineral supplements? The vitamin controversy has been flaming for years. Ever since we learned about the relationship between nutrients and disease, we have wondered if supplements can take the place of or augment food. The facts are that most Americans do not eat the types of foods necessary to ensure optimal amounts of essential vitamins and minerals. Reliance on highly processed products, strict dieting, or high stress lifestyles can inadvertently lead to nutritional deficiencies.

VITAMINS

Vitamins were first recognized as vital to the maintenance of good health in 1906. By 1915, a fat-soluble food factor was extracted from butter, egg yolks, and fish liver, while a water-soluble food factor was extracted from rice bran. In 1920, in order to distinguish the two, the fat-soluble factor was called "vitamin A" and the water-soluble factor "vitamin B." In 1956, more factors were isolated and identified from the original vitamin B "anti-beriberi group," so numbers were added to the letter to further designate them. As other types of vitamins were discovered, they were assigned letters such as vitamins C, D, E, and so on.

What Are Vitamins?

Vitamins are defined as organic (carbon-containing) molecules that are necessary for growth and maintenance of life. Vitamins must be obtained from the foods we eat. An exception to this is vitamin D, which can be obtained from food but more frequently is activated in the skin during exposure to sunlight. Although they are often connected with energy, vitamins provide none themselves but rather speed up the chemical reactions that the body does use for energy.

Vitamins also facilitate the reactions leading to repair and other processes essential to life. The absence of a vitamin will prevent the completion of a reaction, resulting in tissue damage that manifests where the vitamin is most active. For instance, a deficiency of B_2 shows up as cracking at the corners of the mouth and lips, a lack of vitamin A causes night blindness, and a vitamin D deficiency manifests itself as rickets. Prolonged absence of a vitamin may result in a serious illness. Most often, a malfunction involves a number of nutrients instead of one isolated factor since vitamins work together to perform a task. Therefore, the use of complexes or multivitamins may be more beneficial since it can be difficult to isolate the weak links.

Fat-Soluble Vitamins   Vitamins that concentrate in fatty tissues and cell membranes, such as A, D, E, and K, need fat for proper assimilation. On the other hand, because they can be stored in these areas and in the liver, toxic level buildup is possible.

Water-Soluble Vitamins   Vitamins such as B and C are carried by the blood throughout the body and are absorbed by the cells where they are needed. They must be replenished every day from food and, if needed, from supplements because they cannot be stored in the body. Any excess is excreted in the urine although large amounts of an isolated vitamin may create an imbalance if used indiscriminately without adequate knowledge or guidance.

How Much Do We Need?

Supplement labels list the percentage of the U.S. RDA for the particular vitamin within the formula. Since the RDA applies to presumably healthy people, no special considerations are given for people with abnormal metabolic disorders, severe infections, chronic illnesses, certain environmental conditions, or varying lifestyles. Many people can exist on the U.S. RDAs, while others find the vitamin recommendations too low. Higher potencies are warranted for some conditions; substances should be used with discretion and preferably some guidance. Table 8.1 lists some of the more common vitamins. Some are listed without RDAs because of insufficient knowledge about the exact levels needed or because their status as a true vitamin is questioned by the National Academy of Sciences. Dosages for vitamins B, C, and K are expressed in terms of weight, milligrams (mg) or micrograms (mcg), while vitamins A, D, and E are stated in units of activity, international units (i.u.). International units are used with vitamin E instead of milligrams or micrograms to standardize the many forms of E available.

Vitamins As Antioxidants

Among the fastest selling of all vitamins are the antioxidants: vitamins C, E, and beta-carotene. A decade of laboratory research has shown that it is oxidation that makes cholesterol so harmful to coronary arteries. Although only a few human studies have been published, the results indicate that low levels of these vitamins correlate with a higher death rate from heart disease. Findings point to the fact that certain doses of antioxidant supplements can reduce the risk of myocardial infarction by one-half among men with histories of cardiovascular disease. The only side effect found so far is that excessive quantities of vitamin C may cause diarrhea, but since it is water-soluble and expelled in the urine, overdose is not a danger, with the rare exception of the development of renal stones. Vitamin E and beta-carotene can accumulate in our fat stores, but the side effects of this are no more serious than a stomachache or yellowing of the skin, which is reversible with time.

Vitamin and U.S. RDA Level	Function	Food Sources	Deficiency Symptoms
B₁ (Thiamine) 1.5 mg	Needed for carbohydrate digestion, growth in children and maintenance of organ muscle tone. Vital for a healthy nervous system, mental health and linked to improved learning capacity.	Wheat germ, bran, whole grains, blackstrap molasses, nutritional yeast.	Easy fatigue, irritability, loss of appetite, constipation, mental depression.
B₂ (Riboflavin) 1.8 mg	Necessary for cell respiration, food metabolism, maintenance of healthy eyes, skin and mouth.	Liver, tongue, organ meats, egg yolks, milk, cheese, wheat germ.	Cracked lips and corners of mouth, inflammation of mouth, swollen tongue, itching, burning, bloodshot eyes, dizziness, sensitivity to light.
B₃ (Niacin) 20 mg	Acts as a coenzyme in digestion, dilates blood vessels, improves circulation, reduces cholesterol in blood. Needed for healthy skin, proper functioning of nervous system and production of sex hormones.	Lean meats, poultry, fish, peanuts, wheat germ, nutritional yeast.	Muscle weakness, fatigue, insomnia, irritability, canker sores, gastrointestinal disturbances, and recurring headaches.
B₆ (Pyridoxine) 2.0 mg	Needed for production of antibodies and red blood cells, aids digestion, promotes normal functioning of nervous and musculoskeletal systems, reduces cholesterol level in the bloodstream.	Bananas, wheat germ, leafy greens, raw meats, milk.	Low blood sugar, nervousness, hair loss, muscle cramps, water retention and nausea in pregnancy.
Biotin 300 mcg	Metabolism of fats, production of fatty acids, food metabolism and the utilization of other B vitamins.	Found in all animal and plant tissue and traces are present in most whole foods, liver, legumes, egg yolk, meats.	Muscular pain, exhaustion, loss of appetite and depression.
Choline (none stated)	Fat metabolism, cholesterol utilization, normal nerve transmission. Essential for health of liver, kidneys and the production of thyroid hormones.	Wheat germ, lecithin, yeast, egg yolks, liver, whole grains.	Fatty deposits in liver, bleeding ulcers, kidney problems, high blood pressure. Prolonged deficiency can result in cirrhosis of the liver and atherosclerosis.

TABLE 8.1 *Vitamin Information*

Vitamin and U.S. RDA Level	Function	Food Sources	Deficiency Symptoms
Inositol (none stated)	Metabolism of fats and reduction of blood cholesterol, formation of lecithin in the body. Vital for hair growth and brain cell nutrition.	Citrus fruits, whole grains, yeast, liver, milk.	Constipation, eczema, eye problems, hair loss, high blood serum cholesterol.
Folic Acid 400 mcg	Formation of red blood cells, cell growth and reproduction, health of the liver, hair and scalp.	Green leafy vegetables, liver, whole grains, oysters, nutritional yeast.	Gastrointestinal disturbances, hair loss or graying, tongue inflammation, anemia, toxemia in pregnancy.
Pantothenic Acid 10 mg	Stimulation of adrenal glands, utilization of other vitamins, building of body cells, resistance to stress, formation of antibodies and maintenance of normal digestive functions.	Organ meats, egg yolks, nutritional yeast, whole grains, green vegetables, royal jelly.	Digestive problems, hypoglycemia, allergies, upper respiratory infections, burning or tingling feet and skin disorders.
Paba (Para Aminobenzoic Acid) (none stated)	Occurs in combination with folic acid. Promotes red blood cell formation, healthy skin, can restore color to gray hair, creates a natural sunscreen, promotes healthy intestinal flora.	Liver, nutritional yeast, wheat germ, milk, eggs, organ meats, blackstrap molasses.	Constipation and digestive problems, extreme fatigue, headache, loss of hair color and skin pigmentation. Sulfa drugs destroy paba.
B$_{12}$ (Cyanocobalamin) 6 mcg	Construction and regeneration of red blood cells, anti-anemia factor, food metabolism, healthy nervous system.	Liver, meat, fish, milk, eggs, yogurt, miso pollen, wheat germ.	Extreme fatigue, anemia, brain damage, nervous system disorders. Symptoms may take 5 or 6 years to appear.
B$_{15}$ (Pangamic Acid) (none stated)	Promotes cell respiration, antioxidant, regulates fat and sugar metabolism and is essential in protein metabolism, particularly in heart muscle. Stimulates immune responses.	Nutritional yeast, brown rice, whole grains, pumpkin, and sesame seeds.	Glandular and nervous disorders, heart disease.
C 60 mg	Helps prevent infections, strengthens connective tissues, healthy teeth, gums, bones. Promotes healing, maintains integrity of capillaries, collagen production, antioxidant.	Citrus fruits, tomatoes, green peppers, strawberries, kale, broccoli, parsley, most fresh fruits and vegetables.	Bleeding gums, tooth decay, weak capillaries, bruising easily, nosebleeds, lowered resistance to infection, slow healing.

TABLE 8.1 *Vitamin Information (continued)*

Vitamin and U.S. RDA Level	Function	Food Sources	Deficiency Symptoms
A 5,000 i.u.	Insures normal structure and function of cell membranes, acts to fight infection and build disease resistance necessary for healthy skin, bone and teeth formation. Essential for the formation of visual purple, which is necessary for night vision.	Eggs, liver, dairy products, carrots, green leafy vegetables, colored fruits and vegetables.	Night blindness; acne; dry, scaly skin; tooth decay; increased susceptibility to infection.
D 400 i.u.	Proper formation of bones and teeth, thyroid function, normal blood clotting, assimilation of calcium and phosphorus.	Milk, eggs, sardines, salmon, tuna.	Tooth decay, pyorrhea, muscular weakness, porous bones, bone disorders — rickets in children, osteomalacia in adults.
E 30 i.u.	Improves circulation, promotes longevity, antioxidant, prevents blood clots, strengthens capillary walls, aids healing, promotes healthy skin and reproductive organs.	Wheat germ, nuts, seeds, cold pressed vegetable oils, organ meats.	Sterility, miscarriage, heart disease, enlarged prostate, strokes, liver damage.
F (Unsaturated Fatty Acids) (none stated)	Promotes growth, healthy hair and skin, normal glandular activity, destroys cholesterol, helps prevent atherosclerosis, maintains body lubrication.	Butter, wheat germ, vegetable oils, sunflower seeds.	Acne, dandruff, eczema, varicose veins, diarrhea, weak nails, underweight.
K (Phylioquinone) (none stated)	Promotes proper blood clotting, healthy liver function, longevity.	Eggs, soy oil, kelp, yogurt, leafy green vegetables, cauliflower.	Nosebleeds, miscarriages, hemorrhaging due to improper clotting, intestinal malabsorption, diarrhea.
P (Bioflavonoids, Rutin, Hesperidin) (none stated)	Prevents infection, promotes healthy capillary walls and connective tissue, prevents bruising, aids in absorption of vitamin C.	White rind in fruits, cherries, black currants, buckwheat.	Bruising easily, bleeding easily, low resistance to infection, varicose veins.

TABLE 8.1 *Vitamin Information (continued)*

Simply stated, antioxidants work as follows:

1. A normal oxygen atom has four pairs of electrons. Through aging and general wear and tear on our systems, metabolism can take one of the electrons away from the atom. This changes the composition of the oxygen molecule and it becomes a "free radical." This new free radical then attempts to replace its lost electron by attacking other molecules.

2. When the free radical attacks and robs an electron from another molecule in the cell wall, a new free radical is created. A chain reaction begins when this newly created free radical seeks to take an electron from yet another molecule.

3. The chain of electron theft begins to erode the cell membrane and leads to disintegration of the cell. When this occurs, the cell surface is exposed to cancerous changes or a host of other ills.

4. The antioxidants have particular molecular structures. Because of their structure, they can go to the tissue and give up their electrons without becoming harmful and invading other cells. Thus, the chain reaction that culminates in cell-wall disintegration is aborted.

In essence, the antioxidant vitamins C, E, and beta-carotene may control the harmful free radical molecules and thereby prevent many common diseases.

MINERALS

Minerals, one of the most understated classes of nutrients, are finally getting the status they deserve. We are only now beginning to recognize the importance of minerals. For one thing, without minerals, vitamins cannot be assimilated or utilized by the body.

What Are They?

Minerals are used by our bodies to form bones, teeth, soft tissue, muscles, blood, and nerve cells. Besides functioning as structural components, minerals are also catalysts for many reactions within the body, such as transmission of nerve impulses, digestion, and muscle response. In addition, they assist in producing hormones, maintaining the acid/alkaline balance in our bodies, and manufacturing antibodies.

What Foods Have Them?

Highly assimilated organic minerals are found in fruits and vegetables from the soil or sea or from fish or animals whose mineral content originates from eating land or sea plants. A varied diet containing whole grains, beans, nuts and seeds, leafy greens, fruits, and, if desired, dairy products, meat, poultry, fish, and eggs has the potential to provide all the minerals we need. Refined sugars and carbohydrates should be minimized since they retain very few minerals originally present in the food.

How Much Do We Need?

Calcium, chlorine, phosphorus, potassium, magnesium, sodium, and sulfur are called macrominerals because relatively large amounts are needed in the body. Zinc, iron, manganese, copper, chromium, selenium, iodine, and molybdenum are referred to as trace minerals because only minute amounts are required. Although most minerals have a general U.S. RDA established value, trace minerals have a significantly narrow margin of safety. It is easy to take too much, develop toxicity, and create a deficiency in another trace mineral. Unless proper levels of minerals are maintained and monitored, the delicate mineral balance of our bodies can be upset.

Chelated Minerals

Our bodies must convert inorganic minerals from the earth, such as dolomite, oyster shell, egg shell, and bone meal, into an organic form that we can assimilate. A chelated mineral is bound to another substance such as gluconic acid from corn (gluconates), lactic acid from milk or corn (lactates), fumaric acid from plants (fumerates), sulfuric acid (sulfates), ascorbic acid (ascorbates, citric acid, citrates), amino acids from soy or milk protein (amino acid chelates), or orotic acid (oratates).

Table 8.2 details mineral information. Note that some minerals are listed without RDAs because there is insufficient knowledge about the exact levels needed.

VITAMIN AND MINERAL SUPPLEMENTS

Ideally, we should be able to rely on natural foods to supply all the nutrients we need to maintain optimum health. However, where and how the food is grown; how it is processed, transported, and stored; and how old it is when we eat it all affect the nutrient value of food. In addition to the food factors themselves, age, heredity, environment, activity level, stress, and lifestyle determine how we assimilate the nutrients and how much of each one we need.

Common Terms

When reading labels or counseling clients about vitamins and minerals, it is important to know the meaning of the terminology. The following words are commonly used.

Hypoallergenic Denotes that a supplement contains none or few of the foods or substances constituting the most common sensitivities experienced by people. In most cases, the supplement will also be free of artificial flavor, colors, and preservatives.

International units (i.u.) Dosages of vitamins A, D, and E are stated in units of activity rather than weight. International units are used with vitamin E instead of milligrams or micrograms to standardize the many forms of vitamin E available. Their use with vitamins A and D is simply due to historical usage.

Sustained release or timed release supplements These are designed to provide nutrients over a 6- to 12-hour period when frequent doses are not taken. Effectiveness varies with the manufacturer and the digestive system of the person taking the supplement.

Mineral and U.S. RDA Level for adults & children over 4	Function	Food Sources	Deficiency Symptoms
Calcium 800 mg 1,200–1,500 for older women	Builds bones and teeth and maintains bone density and strength. Helps prevent osteoporosis. Plays a role in regulating heartbeat, blood clotting and muscle contraction.	Milk and milk products, sardines and salmon eaten with bones, dark green leafy vegetables, shellfish, sea vegetables, tempeh, rutabagas.	Rickets in children, osteoporosis in adults.
Chloride 700–5,100 mg No RDA established	Maintains normal fluid shifts, balances pH of blood, forms hydrochloric acid in stomach.	Table salt, fish, pickled and smoked foods.	Upset balance of acids and bases in body fluids (RARE)
Chromium 0.03–0.20 mg No RDA established	Important for glucose metabolism, may be a cofactor for insulin.	Meat, cheese, whole grains, dried peas and beans, peanuts, brewer's yeast.	Diabeteslike symptoms.
Copper 2 mg No RDA established	Formation of red blood cells, cofactor in absorbing iron into blood, helps in production of several enzymes involved in respiration, interacts with zinc.	Organ meats, shellfish, nuts, dried legumes, raisins, mushrooms.	Rarely seen in adults. Infants: hypochronic anemia with abnormal development of bone, nervous tissue, lungs and pigmentation of hair.
Fluorine 1–4.0 mg No RDA established	Contributes to solid bone and tooth formation; may help prevent osteoporosis in adults.	Naturally or artificially fluoridated water, some kinds of black tea.	Higher frequency of tooth decay.
Iodine 0.15 mg	Necessary for normal function of thyroid gland, essential for normal cell function, prevents goiter.	Sea vegetables, iodized salt, seafood, plants grown in iodine-rich soil.	Thyroid enlargement (goiter) Newborns: cretinism.
Iron 10 mg (male) 18 mg (female)	Essential to formation of hemoglobin —the oxygen-carrying factor in the blood—and myoglobin—which stores oxygen in muscles.	Liver, meat products, egg yolk, shellfish, green leafy vegetables, legumes, whole grains, dried fruits.	Iron deficiency anemia, pallor of skin, weakness and fatigue, headache, shortness of breath.
Magnesium 200–300 mg	Aids in bone growth, nerve conduction, muscle relaxation, regulation of normal heart rhythm, bowel function.	Nuts, legumes, whole grains, bananas, apricots, dark leafy greens.	Muscular tremors, twitching, and weakness. Deficiency is sometimes seen in people with severe disease, prolonged diarrhea, or alcoholism.

TABLE 8.2   Mineral Information

Mineral and U.S. RDA Level for adults & children over 4	Function	Food Sources	Deficiency Symptoms
Manganese 1.5–5.0 mg	Required for normal bone growth and development, part of some enzymes.	Nuts, whole grains, legumes, non-leafy vegetables, fruits, tea.	Not well defined in humans.
Molybdenum 0.06–5.0 mg No RDA established	Enzyme constituent.	Whole grains, legumes, organ meats, dark green vegetables.	Unknown in humans.
Phosphorus 800 mg	With calcium helps build strong bones and teeth. Needed by certain enzymes that help change food into energy.	Meat, poultry, fish, eggs, legumes, milk and milk products, whole grains.	Weakness, bone pain, neurological problems (RARE).
Potassium 775–5,624 mg	With sodium helps regulate body-fluid balance, transmission of nerve impulses, active in muscle contraction, promotes regular heartbeat.	Most fruits, starchy root vegetables, dark leafy green vegetables, peanut butter.	Muscular weakness, irritability, irregular heartbeat.
Selenium 0.03–0.20 mg No RDA established	Cellular antioxidant, essential constituent of red blood cells, enzymes, decreases the toxicity of heavy metals, may inhibit cancer initiation.	Fish, shellfish, chicken, egg yolks, garlic, whole grains.	Heart muscle damage, hemolytic anemia.
Sodium 450–3,300 mg No RDA established	Helps maintain water balance inside and outside cells, plays a role in maintaining blood pressure.	Salt, processed foods, ham, pickles, smoked foods.	Muscle weakness, cramps, confusion, apathy, anorexia, low blood pressure.
Zinc 10–15 mg	Essential for more than 100 enzymes involved in growth, sexual maturation, wound healing, ability to taste, protein synthesis, immunity.	Meats, eggs, oysters, crabmeat, nuts, wheat germ.	Loss of taste, delayed wound healing, growth retardation and delayed sexual maturation in children.

TABLE 8.2 *Mineral Information (continued)*

U.S. Recommended Dietary Allowance (U.S. RDA)   Estimates established by the Federal Drug Administration (FDA) to ensure against deficiencies in healthy people.

Vegetarian supplements   Supplements that are free of any animal products or derivatives. They are sold as tablets, powders, or liquids; capsules are usually avoided because of beef gelatin source.

Natural Versus Synthetic

A truly natural supplement is one that is a concentrated food source. Vitamins A and D are natural if they are derived from fish liver oil, alfalfa, rose hips, brewer's yeast, wheat germ oil, lecithin, or desiccated liver. Natural vitamin E sources are soy oil, bone meal, chlorophyll, aloe vera, evening primrose oil, and spirulina. However, many supplements are derived from a synthetic source, a laboratory product whose molecular structure is similar to the supplement being copied. Synthetic supplements are used because of the advantages of synthetic over natural in terms of cost, availability of a natural commercial source, size limitations on the pill itself, and the number of pills required for a certain potency.

Vitamins from a natural source can be concentrated only to a certain degree. Most B and C supplements are at least partially synthetic to provide quantities that can be used to offset a deficiency. However, it is possible to concentrate high potencies of vitamins A, D, and E from the natural sources. Natural sources can be beneficial because they may contain synergistic elements, naturally occurring coenzymes, and other vitamins and minerals that facilitate assimilation in our bodies. Many companies add a natural base to their synthetic supplements in order to provide the best results. In contrast, some people prefer to use pure synthetic supplements to avoid natural substances to which they are allergic or sensitive.

Both natural-source and synthetic-source supplements work well. Vitamin E is the only vitamin that is definitely recognized to be more effective in the natural state. Personal preference and the potency required are the determining factors in choosing a natural or synthetic supplement. If you require only minimal amounts to supplement your diet, natural supplements may be suitable. If you need higher potencies to offset a deficiency or if you have food sensitivities, you may want a synthetic-based supplement.

How Much Do We Need?

With a good foundation of a balanced diet, plenty of exercise, and adequate sleep, supplements can be an effective booster if more nutrients are actually needed. However, without test results and professional guidance, it is difficult to know what and how much to take. Pregnant and lactating women, heavy drinkers, women on oral contraceptives, and those who are unable to get an adequate diet due to a prolonged illness, digestive disorders, physical or emotional problems, or dieting can find it difficult to get all the nutrients they need from food. In these cases, supplements are beneficial.

Using the standards of the U.S. RDAs as general guidelines, many people start with a low-potency multiple vitamin/mineral supplement to cover most of the available nutrients in a balanced ratio. Keep in mind that more is not always better. The toxicity symptoms of a nutrient are sometimes similar to the deficiency symptoms and isolated doses of one nutrient may cause an imbalance. Higher potencies are warranted for some conditions, but they should be used with discretion and preferably under guidance.

When and How to Take Supplements

Fat-soluble supplements should be taken with foods to enhance absorption and to prevent nausea. If taken once a day, take them with the largest meal, preferably earlier in the day to avoid the stimulation that sometimes interferes with sleep. Water-soluble vitamins can be taken between meals. Calcium with meals may deplete the level of stomach acidity necessary for proper digestion; therefore, consider taking calcium between meals and at bedtime.

Storage

Without preservation, supplements will keep 2 to 3 years if the bottle is unopened. Once opened, they will keep up to 1 year. Store in a cool, dry place away from sunlight. Do not store in the refrigerator because moisture builds up inside the bottle after constant opening and closing. Some companies add a silica gel packet to absorb excess moisture. A few grains of rice added to the bottle will give similar results.

Forms of Supplements

Supplements are available in many forms to facilitate the particular absorption requirements of the various nutrients and to provide alternatives for individual needs and desires.

Tablets   These are the most familiar form and are easily stored. They usually require the addition of fillers and binders to form the tablet from loose material. High-pressure compression and coatings protect the tablets from moisture and facilitate swallowing. Some tablets are so compact that some people may have difficulty with absorption and utilization.

Chewable Tablets   These are most often sweetened with sugar, honey, molasses, fructose, or fruit concentrates. They are easy to take and are generally well-absorbed. The sugar content can be quite high, so if sugar is to be avoided, use powders, liquids, or capsules.

Powders and Liquids   These forms are very well-assimilated and are usually quite potent. They can be mixed into liquids, foods, or taken by the spoonful. Unpalatable combinations generally are sweetened or flavored.

Capsules   These are usually well-assimilated, easy to swallow, and tasteless. Capsules are not suitable for strict vegetarians because they are made from animal gelatin. Vegetarians and those who are allergic to beef can open the capsule, swallow the contents, and discard the capsule.

SUMMARY

We have learned a great deal about vitamins and minerals since they were first recognized at the beginning of this century. Understanding their importance as we now do, we should ascertain our own needs and our clients' needs for adequate vitamin intake. Knowing that length of time of body storage varies from one vitamin to another, we should maintain a diet filled with nutritious foods.

Suggested Reading

Somer, E. (1992). *The essential guide to vitamins and minerals.* New York: HarperCollins Publishers.
Ulene, A., & Ulene, V. (1994). *The vitamin strategy.* Berkeley, CA: Ulysses Press.

9 EMOTIONS AND FOOD

OVERVIEW

We all know the power of emotions. Sometimes they consume us, and sometimes we have them under control, but they are always with us. How we deal with the relationship between food and emotions is a significant part of who we are and how we respond.

CASE STUDY | *Sarah*

Sarah sat with her knee skinned and her head throbbing. She had fallen off her bicycle again. Soon Mother came out to hold and cuddle her and to put a bandage on that little cut—and to give her an ice cream cone to cheer her up.

Twenty years later, Sarah's pride is skinned and her head is throbbing. In the last year, she has gone through a divorce, been in a car accident, and lost her job. On top of all of this, she has gained nearly 40 pounds.

THE INTERTWINING RELATIONSHIP

Food and emotions are intertwined. From the time we are children, we are taken out to dinner for rewards, served ice cream when we hurt, and given pizza to celebrate. Virtually all of our happy holidays are filled with food. We have, in essence, become a society where food is all important. Who has ever heard of a social gathering without the hors d'oeuvres or Thanksgiving with just laughter and happiness and no turkey and dressing? We probably cannot imagine having a really happy time without food being included in some way. Even when we go to the movies, we are tempted by popcorn and candy.

As we consider the relationship between emotions and food, let us look at Sarah as an example. When Sarah was a child and was hurt and given ice cream, she felt much better. Why? Because ice cream was a special treat, something that her mother gave her to prove that even with her knee hurting, ice cream could still taste good. Falling off her bike did not mean that she was a failure. To prove it, she was given a reward.

Twenty years later, Sarah is still a good person. To prove that to herself, despite the failed marriage, she rewards herself with lots of delicious foods. Thus, a vicious cycle begins. The causative emotions in this instance are sadness and hurt. This probably results in reduced self-esteem. Going through a divorce is hard, but making herself a big plate of steaming hot, high-calorie food not only reassures Sarah, it is also delicious and warm. With this meal, she can tell herself that even though she did not succeed in her marriage or in her job, food still tastes good.

CASE STUDY | *Larry*

Larry jumped up and laughed. He had just received one of the top Scholastic Aptitude Test (SAT) scores in the nation. His parents, who were proud and happy for him, took him out to dinner where he ate his fill with a smile on his lips. Later when he got accepted into medical school, his parents threw him a dinner party one night, and he and his friends celebrated with pizza the next.

Ten years later, Larry is getting sued for malpractice. His wife and children stand by him supportingly, but nothing seems to help. He knows that he has done nothing wrong; he has done his best. Despite how he tries, he cannot bring himself to have even a bite of the wonderful dinner his wife has prepared for him. He can tell she is worried about his weight loss during the past month, but somehow he feels much too sad to even touch his food. What if the malpractice suit goes to court?

Observation

For his whole life, Larry has used food as a reward. When he was happy he ate, when he won something he ate, when things where going well he was able to eat. Yet, when he most needs the vitamins and minerals in food, he cannot even bring himself to touch it.

Emotional Links

We know that there is a link between emotions and food. We need food to live, not just physically it seems, but emotionally. If we are at a comfortable weight, there is nothing wrong with rewarding ourselves with an occasional treat. Some of us, though, need food to feel happy or reassured.

Food is our psychologist. The problem, however, is that this food "psychologist" can cause trouble when we go to it for reassurance, as Sarah and Larry found. In Sarah's case, it caused her to put on weight. This made her feel more depressed, which led her to eat again. In Larry's case, he ate when he was succeeding or doing well, but when he really needed food, he rejected it.

Indulging ourselves occasionally if we are happy and maintain a healthy weight is fine, but food can become a problem when we link it too heavily with emotions.

___

ANGER

Anger is an emotion that we have all experienced.

CASE STUDY | *Tina*

While I was preparing to attend a dinner party, I got a frantic call from my friend, Tina. She was out-of-breath and upset because her son had taken their car without telling her, and she had no way to get to the party. We agreed that my husband and I would pick her up.

Tina looked good; she was wearing black to downplay the weight she had gained in the last year. As Tina talked, I could tell she was furious. Her son had been staying out late and his grades were falling. When we sat down for dinner, Tina attacked her food.

After dinner, we drove Tina home. Her son had arrived home by then. I walked her to the door and she seemed much calmer. When she saw her son, she politely said that there was something they needed to discuss. Then they both sat down at the table, and I left. Later she told me that she had behaved calmly and rationally and that she and the boy had come up with a system for sharing the car.

The point of this story is to see the connection between anger and food. Tina ripped her chicken entrée to shreds, devoured two baked potatoes, three helpings of green beans, and two pieces of cheesecake. She seemingly took her anger out on the food by eating it. Later, with a full stomach, she used her calmness with her son. She had previously learned that her anger with him did not get her anywhere except back to the refrigerator.

Observation

Anger is a very primitive emotion, yet we still need it. Anger should motivate us to take action. It should not cause us to pick up the phone and call for a pizza. For Tina, it should have let her know that she needed help with her son. She should have used her anger to ground him or to find a really good place to hide the car keys. Anger should be used to benefit us, not to cause a weight problem.

HATE

Hate and anger are strongly related and often cause the same problems.

CASE STUDY | *Carol*

My daughter has a friend named Carol who is a little plump. She is also very intelligent. One day we all went out for pizza as a reward for their good grades. During our meal, Carol told me about a girl who she strongly disliked, mainly because her boyfriend had left her to date the other girl. While Carol talked about the girl, I noticed that Carol was eating very fast. She consumed half of our large pizza while she was talking about her hate/anger towards this girl and her boyfriend.

Observation

For a nation so obsessed with food, it is incredible to observe how much injurious emotion we lend to it. Both Carol and Tina took out their negative emotions by devouring as much food as possible.

LOVE

Now that we have talked about two negative emotions, let us consider a positive one, love. Love and food are quite a combination. Most of the time when people first fall in love the desire to eat is not very strong. Why? Because deep down our bodies know they would rather reproduce than have a piece of cheesecake. As time goes on, however, love turns more to companionship, and we enjoy sharing our meals with our partners. When we eat together, we need to help each other by picking out healthy foods. Then we can go home, cuddle up, and have some fun working off the calories together.

Love is an emotion we often feel for others but not enough for ourselves, especially concerning what we eat. If we really cared about ourselves, we would want to stay healthy by exercising and eating low-fat foods. The most important part of the emotion love is learning to feel it about ourselves.

HAPPINESS

Happiness is a positive emotion, but we do not gain or lose weight because we are happy or sad. We create weight problems when we use food to satisfy our emotions, to reward ourselves, to relieve stress, or to vent. When we allow our untethered emotions to rule us, some of us starve ourselves, while others become obese.

Let us refer back to Larry. Larry is basically a happy person, someone who loves a good meal. Yet with any sadness, he loses his will to eat. Larry is the type of person who does not care if food still tastes good, because his life is in torment. Larry still needs to eat, but food and emotion have become so linked in him that when he is unhappy, he loses his desire to eat.

In good times or in bad, we need to treat ourselves well. Take a long bath, see a good movie, and indulge in an occasional banana split. But just make sure the banana split includes a banana, and some low-fat frozen yogurt, and is topped with only a small portion of chocolate sauce. After the treat, take a walk and resolve the issue. By working with our emotions, we can benefit ourselves, not the local pizza parlor.

THE IMPORTANCE OF HOW WE EAT

How we eat is as important as what we eat. Many of us rush through our meals, gulping our food while paying little or no attention to what we are eating. We may be distracted by television, conversation, reading, or even daydreaming during our meals. The point is that we are not paying attention to our food. More often than not, when we eat like this, we gain weight, especially around mid-life.

Many religious orders, both Western and Eastern, teach the importance of mindful eating. Mindful eating requires us to pay attention to what, with whom, how, when, where, and why we are eating. The theory behind mindful eating is that when we pause to reflect on the source, the preparation, the texture, the color, the shape, the arrangement, and so forth of the food item before us, we will better appreciate its value. As we consider the value of the food, we consider other aspects of its assimilation; for example, of what benefit is this food to us? How will this food make us stronger, healthier, or better able to perform? There is no question that these reflective questions will better bind us to the food we eat and put us in a position to seriously consider what we are doing to and with our bodies. Attention to these questions constitutes the beginning phase of mindful eating.

To facilitate this exercise, begin by eating alone. Turn off the television and seat yourself in a comfortable setting. Examine the foods before you and think about the holistic aspects of each food item while you eat it. Calm your emotions. Think about the chewing process. Feel the foods and consider their effect on your body. As you practice this technique, notice how as you increase your attention to the food, you both decrease your speed and calm yourself.

After you have done this exercise alone a few times, try it in a group setting. It's best to begin with your family. Perhaps you will want to involve them in the process. You will probably notice that your speed of eating has slowed compared to others. As you gain skill in mindful eating, you will find that you can even eat mindfully in a group. You will probably find, however, that you are a little slower and probably calmer than your friends. Just remember, the idea is to completely nourish your body, mind, and spirit. Doing this requires mindfulness.

SUMMARY

Food and emotions are interrelated, but they need not be directly correlated to the extent that they rule our lives. Each day and every event gives us opportunities to respond with positive, negative, and/or neutral emotions and to develop emotional self-control. Emotional balance can be achieved with conscious effort. When we discipline our emotions and achieve emotional harmony, we are in a superior position to develop healthy eating behaviors. One of the keys to vibrant health is to develop eating habits based on sensible, conscious choices rather than on the dictates of unconscious emotional drives.

Suggested Reading

Billigmeier, S. (1991). *Inner eating: How to free yourself forever from the tyranny of food.* Nashville, TN: Oliver-Nelson Books.

Greeson, J., (1993). *Food for love, healing the food, sex, love, and intimacy relationship.* New York: Simon and Schuster.

Greeson, J. (1993). *It's not what you're eating, it's what's eating you.* New York: Simon and Schuster.

Hirschmann, J., & Munter, C. (1988). *Overcoming eating.* New York: Ballantine Books.

Hollis, J. (1994). *Fat and furious.* New York: Ballantine Books.

Roth, G. (1991). *When food is love.* New York: Penguin Books.

NUTRITION
THROUGH
THE LIFESPAN

Nutritional needs vary throughout the lifespan. This chapter focuses on the differences that occur during the developmental and receding years.

YOUTH

Infants

Milk is the first food for infants. It is now generally accepted that the mother's breast milk is the food of choice for babies from birth to weaning. Weaning age varies from person to person and culture to culture. For most babies, it is between 6 months to 1 year of age.

Formula-fed babies follow the specific regimens prescribed by their practitioners. Following the switch from formula to regular milk, it is important that skim milk not be used for infants. Skim milk lacks linoleic acid (essential fatty acid) and has inadequate calories.

Introduction of solid foods should not begin until at least after 2 to 3 months of age because salivary amylase for the digestion of starches is not present until then. Cereals are usually introduced first. If the sweeter fruits are introduced first, the baby will reject the cereal in preference of the sweeter taste. Egg whites should not be offered until the baby is over 12 months because infants frequently develop allergies to the protein in egg whites before this age.

Preschool Children

Children from 1 to 3 years of age slow their rate of growth from that of infancy. They have a decreased appetite and consequent decrease in food consumption. During this time, they manifest a desire for independence and often will favor non-nutritious foods. From 3 to 6 years their requirements do not change much, but this is the time they observe others for eating habits and styles. If the parents eat nutritious foods, the child will probably follow. On the other hand, if the parents are fast-food junkies, the preschool-age child will likely emulate this style.

School-Age Children

From 6 to 12 years, children grow slowly and steadily. Continued protein intake is important for muscle development, and milk intake is important for bone development. At this age, vitamin A and C deficiencies are common because many children do not have an adequate intake of the recommended quantities of fresh fruits and vegetables.

Adolescence

Between the ages of 12 and 20, the rate of growth is greater than at any other period of life except infancy. Girls may add over 3 inches, and boys 4 or more inches in height. Because of this growth spurt, the need for calories will increase at some time during this period. Boys may need 2,700 to 2,900 calories per day, and girls will require 2,100 to 2,200 calories per day.

During this period, it is important to maintain sufficient protein intake. Boys need protein for the development of muscle mass and long bone growth, which are controlled by testosterone. Girls need protein for the synthesis of increased fat tissues and long bone growth.

The need for the minerals calcium and phosphorus is 50 percent higher than it is during childhood because of the increased bone growth. Iron is particularly important in girls to replace what is lost during menstruation and in boys for muscle development. Of course, all other vitamins and minerals must be consumed at the recommended levels.

ADULTS

Adults will want to adhere to the principles presented throughout this book. The one variation of adulthood not mentioned in other sections of this book is the special needs of athletes. Adult athletes differ from nonathletes in their nutritional requirements. A balanced diet for athletes consists of 60 percent of calories from carbohydrates, 15 percent from protein, and 25 percent from fat. Other important considerations include adequate intake of minerals and fluids (Holt, 1993). Energy needs of ultraendurance athletes during training vary widely, depending upon duration, intensity, and type of exercise training. It is not known whether protein needs are increased in ultraendurance athletes as a result of extended exercise training. Micronutrient needs may be altered for these athletes while dietary intake is generally over the RDA because of high caloric intake. Prior to competition, ultraendurance athletes should consider glycogen supercompensation and a prerace meal eaten 4 hours before the race as a means of improving performance (Applegate, 1991). Most athletes do not have dietary deficiencies, but those who restrict their food intake in order to maintain body weight are more likely to be deficient in folate, B_6, B_{12}, and E. Some female athletes' diets are low in calcium, iron, and zinc. Low calcium intake may reduce peak bone mass in young women (Haymes, 1991).

ELDERS

Demographics

As we race into the future, we Americans will be showing our age. The elderly population is the fastest growing segment in the United States today. Demographers estimate that by the year 2,000, one in four of us will be over 65. The fastest growing segment of old people are those now classified as the old-old, elders over 85. The challenge for us, as nurses, is to reach out to our burgeoning elderly population and guide them in the whys and wherefores of healing nutrition before they succumb to the preventable ravages of faulty nutrition.

CASE STUDY | *Mike*

Mike, an 87-year-old retired executive, lived in an exclusive apartment building in an elite section of a major city. The widower had two daughters, aged 60 and 64, who lived with their children in an adjoining state and seldom visited, and a successful son nearing retirement in a distant state. Mike had an income of $2,600 a month and a quarter of a million dollars in assets, yet he was starving to death. Neither his remaining few friends nor his relatives realized he was subsisting on over-the-counter coffee cakes and root beers.

Mike arose each day at 6:00 A.M., brewed a pot of coffee, and lounged through the morning reading the paper and working on his investment accounts. In the late morning, he went out to a local cafe and ordered the breakfast pastry of the day, usually a wedge of high-fat, high-sugar coffee cake. On most days, he had another cup of coffee to wash down the pastry and then strolled through the park and shop fronts making his way home around 1:00 P.M.

He knew that a local senior center offered midday meals, but he had a prejudice against that group. He thought only low-income people went there. Also, he had become quite antisocial since the death of his wife two years ago. During the afternoon, he tinkered with model cars, a hobby he had never had time for during his working years. More often than not, he took a nap during his hobby afternoons. When he awoke, he liked to have a frosty root beer. He kept a good stock in his kitchen. At 6:00 P.M., he turned on the television and usually flipped channels and watched programs while he resumed work on his model cars and drank from his stock of root beer.

On weekends, one of his children would call or he would call them. On holidays, he usually traveled to one of their homes and stayed a night or two. He ate sparsely since his stomach had shrunk and his appetite waned. No one particularly noticed, and no changes occurred. It was not until two years later, when a much older, feeble Mike fell and sprained his ankle that anyone paid any attention to his health.

At the emergency department of the city hospital, the staff decided to admit Mike for observation. After he was admitted, an intake assessment was done. At this time, it became apparent that Mike was suffering from malnutrition related to inadequate intake. Skin lesions, emaciation, and muscle wasting were among the overt external signs. The internal changes would also have to be assessed and corrected. Both would require time, effort, money, and reeducation.

Observation

This widower is representative of millions like him. As we move into the next century, there are going to be increasing numbers of people like Mike, elders who, while trying to adjust to the changes of old age, forget the importance of eating. Economic status is not a factor in geriatric malnutrition; it can happen to any elder left alone. Geriatric nursing offers an area of specialization that is becoming increasingly meaningful as we have growing numbers of people who need the attention of nurses to guide them into a graceful, fulfilling, healthy old age.

Older Adults Nutrition Facts

Energy expenditure and caloric intake typically decline with age. As nutrient and caloric intake decline, a parallel decline in vitamin and mineral intake is inevitable (Kerstetter, Holthausen, & Fitz, 1993). A contributing factor is that many elderly people live alone and often do not bother to cook for themselves. The result is that many mature adults do not enjoy food as much as they did. Many must literally make themselves sit down and eat meals. Consequently, they tend to eat more comfort foods, such as puddings, cakes, and cookies. Unfortunately sweet foods do not provide the nutrients they need.

Currently, RDAs for those age 51 years and older are extrapolated from younger adult population groups. The recommended caloric intake for seniors is roughly 16 percent less than that advised for other adults. For men between 51 and 75 years, nutritionists generally recommend consuming about 2,400 calories a day. Active elders can consume more calories.

There is strong evidence that aging affects the requirements for certain vitamins. The 1989 Recommended Dietary Allowances appear to be too low for elderly people for vitamin D, riboflavin, vitamin B_6, and vitamin B_{12}, and too high for vitamin A (Russell & Suter, 1993). Deficiencies or suboptimal intakes of water-soluble vitamins, vitamin D, calcium, zinc, copper, chromium, and water are reported in groups of older adults. Marginal nutrient deficiencies in this population may easily go undetected and contribute to morbidity (Kerstetter, Holthausen, & Fitz, 1993).

The RDA of proteins for older people is 12 percent to 15 percent of total calories. The calcium requirement is 800 milligrams, which is equal to about 3 cups of milk. Recommendations for older people aim at correcting or preventing deficiencies by use of supplementary and complementary nutritional products (Vellas et al., 1992).

Many elderly people have trouble eating or swallowing because of tooth pain or ill-fitting dentures. Many live on low or fixed incomes, and some take medications that cause adverse nutrient interactions. Their appetites may be reduced, their senses of taste and smell may be impaired, or they may suffer from chronic diseases. All of these factors contribute to the declining nutritional status of our valued senior citizens. By increasing our awareness of these facts and by knowing that increasing numbers of people like Mike will be needing nursing services, we will be in a better position to discover ways to better serve this population.

SUMMARY

Our bodies are constantly changing. Our 400 billion cells develop, grow, die, and are shed continuously. During active stages of life, we need micronutrients and calories in greater quantities than during other, more quiescent, stages of life. It behooves us, as nurses, to be aware of these differences so that we can better assist all people in healing nutrition.

References

Applegate, E. A. (1991). Nutritional considerations for ultraendurance performance. *International Journal of Sport Nutrition, 1*(2), 118–126.

Haymes, E. M. (1991). Vitamin and mineral supplementation to athletes. *International Journal of Sports Nutrition, 1*(2), 146–169.

Holt, W. S. (1993). Nutrition and athletes. *American Family Physician, 47*(8) 1757–1764.

Kerstetter, J. E., Holthausen, B. A., & Fitz, P.A. (1993). Nutrition and nutritional requirements for the older adult. *Dysphagia, 8*(1), 51–58.

Russell, R. M., & Suter, P. M. (1993). Vitamin requirements of elderly people: An update. *American Journal of Clinical Nutrition, 58*(1), 4–14.

Vellas, B., Grancher, A., Adoue, D., Lafont, C., Fontan, B., & Albarede, J. (1992). Dietary intake recommended for elderly persons. *Presse Medicale, 21*(12), 574–579.

NEW DIMENSIONS OF HEALING FOODS

11 | NEW FOOD FACTS

FOOD LABELING

New food labeling laws went into effect in 1994. Prior to the advent of the new labels, the nutritional content of processed foods was a mystery to grocery store customers. Due to consumer legislation, food products now require generic labels in order that shoppers can make an intelligent choice when selecting foods from supermarket shelves. Each processed food item must carry a label detailing selected nutritional facts. The label begins with serving size and number of servings per container, followed by amount of calories per serving, including how many of these calories come from fat. The next area lists total fat, cholesterol, sodium, a breakdown of carbohydrates, and protein. The percentages of vitamins and minerals are listed next.

Foods Not Covered

Not every food item is required to carry the new label. Raw, single-ingredient meat and poultry products, fresh fish, and 20 of the most popular fruits and vegetables do not have to comply. Other exempt items include foods served in restaurants, purchased in delicatessens, sold in small packages, or produced by small businesses. Other exceptions to the nutritional panel format are allowed on labels of foods made specifically for children under the age of 4 because the FDA has not established daily values for this age group.

Reading the Label

The new food labels should contribute greatly to savvy shoppers' diets. By carefully reading and comparing labels, consumers can make healthy choices in food selection. For example, when comparing labels you might be surprised to learn that a can of soup has 35 calories of fat per serving, while a serving of baked snack chips has only 30 calories from fat. On the same label, we read that the soup has 7 percent of the daily value of cholesterol, while the snack chips have no cholesterol. If you have not yet begun the practice of label reading, start now. You will be amazed at the difference it can make in controlling your nutrient intake. Figure 11.1 illustrates the label and how to read it.

THE FOOD PYRAMID

Most nurses know about the pyramid conceptualized by Abraham Maslow in his theory of the hierarchy of human needs. The principle in Maslow's pyramid is that we need to meet basic physiologic needs before advancing to the apex of self-actualization. Since the pyramid concept is easy to grasp, food theorists have come up with a new one, the food guide pyramid. This pyramid is a general guide that outlines what we need to eat each day to maintain basic requirements. The illustrations of the four food groups and the food group wheel that were used in general and professional education for so long are obsolete. In April of 1992, the U.S. Department of Agriculture (USDA), with the endorsement of the U.S. Department of Health and Human Services (DHHS) issued the food guide pyramid to illustrate the new food categories.

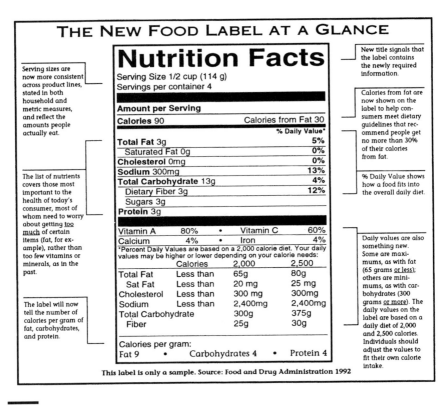

FIGURE 11.1 **The new food label at a glance.**

Source: Food and Drug Administration, 1992.

At the base of the pyramid are foods that come from grains. The bulk of our intake should come from this area. These foods supply fiber, complex carbohydrates, vitamins, and minerals. The second level represents fruits and vegetables. Foods from plants supply multiple and diverse nutrient needs. The third level includes meat, poultry, fish, dry beans, eggs, and nuts. These are important sources of protein, iron, and zinc. Adjacent to this group is the milk, yogurt, and cheese group. Calcium and protein are the primary nutrients in this group. Less protein foods are necessary than vegetables and fruits. The small tip of the pyramid represents fats, oils, and sweets. This group includes salad dressings, oils, butter, margarine, cream, soft drinks, candy, and sweet desserts. These foods provide calories but little else nutritionally. Figure 11.2 depicts the food pyramid.

Food Guide Pyramid
A Guide to Daily Food Choices

KEY

● Fat (naturally occurring and added)   ▼ Sugars (added)

These symbols show fats, oils, and added sugars in foods.

Fats, Oils, & Sweets
USE SPARINGLY

Milk, Yogurt, & Cheese Group
2-3 SERVINGS

Meat, Poultry, Fish, Dry Beans, Eggs, & Nuts Group
2-3 SERVINGS

Vegetable Group
3-5 SERVINGS

Fruit Group
2-4 SERVINGS

Bread, Cereal, Rice, & Pasta Group
6-11 SERVINGS

FIGURE 11.2   *The food guide pyramid.*

Source: U.S. Department of Agriculture and the U.S. Department of Health and Human Services. Provided by the Education Department of the National Live Stock and Meat Board.

One of the hallmarks of the food pyramid guide is that it is based on a recommended number of servings for each of the levels on the pyramid. Serving sizes are shown in table 11.1. If you eat a larger portion, it gets counted as an additional serving. For example, 1/2 cup of cooked pasta counts as one serving in the bread group. If you eat one cup of pasta, that counts as two servings. If you eat a smaller portion, count it as part of a serving. Use servings as a general guide. For mixed foods, estimate the food group serving of the main ingredients. For example, a large slice of pizza counts in the bread group (crust), the milk group (cheese), and the vegetable group (tomato sauce). A cup size helping of beef stew counts as one serving of meat and one serving of vegetables.

Food Item	Amount in Serving
Bread, cereal, rice, pasta	1 oz. ready-to-eat cereal
	1/2 cup cooked cereal, rice, or pasta
	1 slice of bread
	1/2 bagel or hamburger bun
Vegetable	1 cup raw, leafy vegetables
	1/2 cup other vegetables, cooked or raw
	3/4 cup of vegetable juice
Fruit	1/2 cup of cooked or canned fruit
	1 medium apple, banana, or orange
	3/4 cup of fruit juice
Milk, yogurt, or cheese	1 cup milk or yogurt
	1½ oz. natural cheese
	2 oz. processed cheese
Meat, poultry, fish,	1/2 cup cooked dry beans
beans, eggs, and nuts	1 egg
	2–3 oz. cooked lean meat, poultry, or fish
	4 tbs. peanut butter

TABLE 11.1   *Food Serving Sizes*

Table 11.2 gives samples of how many servings from each group are recommended for each of the calorie categories. The calorie category allocations are discussed in chapter 4, Basic Nutritional Needs.

The food pyramid is easy to understand and fun to follow. Instead of thinking of foods in four groups, reorient your thinking to pyramids.

Food Group	1,600 Calories	2,200 Calories	2,800 Calories
Bread group servings	6	9	11
Vegetable group servings	3	4	5
Fruit group servings	2	3	4
Milk group servings	2–3*	2–3*	2–3*
Meat group (in ounces)	5**	6**	7
Total fat (in grams)	53	73	93
Added sugars (in tsp.)+	6	12	18

* Young adults 18 to 24 years old need 3 servings. Teenagers 11 to 18 years and pregnant women need 4 servings. Lactating women need 5 servings.

** Pregnant women need 6 ounces per day and lactating women need 7 to 8 ounces of meat per day.

+ Added from candy, desserts, soft drinks, and other sweets.

TABLE 11.2   *Suggested Daily Servings Based on Caloric Needs*

THE MEDITERRANEAN DIET PYRAMID

The most recent and still controversial nutrition plan to emerge is the Mediterranean Diet Pyramid. The new Mediterranean diet proposal was created by a team of nutritionists and epidemiologists from the World Health Organization (WHO) and Harvard's School of Public Health. The team spent two years devising this new plan as a response to the USDA food guide pyramid. Their goal was to emulate those parts of the Mediterranean region that in the recent past have enjoyed the lowest recorded rates of chronic disease and the highest adult life expectancy. The proposal features its own pyramid along with recommendations for consuming one or two glasses of wine a day and engaging in physical activity (Miller, 1994). See figure 11.3.

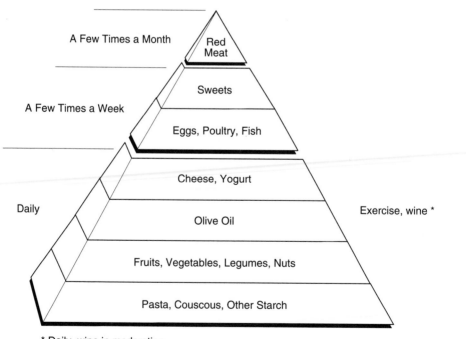

FIGURE 11.3   Mediterranean diet pyramid.

The call for the daily dose of wine adds new heat to one of the biggest controversies in public health today. Growing evidence suggests that wine plays a role in protecting against heart disease, but only when consumed in moderation. The problem, of course, is that many people use more than recommended. Thus, from a contemporary public health perspective, wine should be considered optional. The new plan was introduced in the United States during the summer of 1994.

SUMMARY

Within the past few years, we have witnessed dramatic changes in the organization and description of approaches to healthy eating. The Food Pyramid and the Mediterranean Diet Pyramid detail new dietary recommendations for the American public, while new food labels guide us in selecting individual food products. When following the pyramid approaches, we will eat less meaty protein and increase fruits, grains, and complex carbohydrates. Some of us may prefer to choose the Mediterranean diet regime and include more olive oils and a daily glass of wine.

Reference

Miller, M. W. (1994, June 17). Call for a daily dose of wine ferments critics. *The Wall Street Journal,* pp. B1–2.

12 LIVING FOODS

Some nutritionists believe that the closer food is to the living state, the better. The primary reason for this is that living foods contain living enzymes, which are the building blocks of cells. Most foods, despite their freshness, have been separated from their earth source and hence have begun the decaying process. Although it may be days, weeks, or in some cases months before the food deteriorates completely, nutrients begin the fading process immediately following harvest. The longer the time span from the reaping stage to the consumption stage, the greater the deterioration. Also, the greater the degree of processing the greater the amount of nutrient loss.

Some foods are still in a living state when we consume them. Yogurt and sprouted seeds are among the foods available to us in the living state. Salads and dishes made from fresh fruits and vegetables are the best known living foods.

SPROUTED SEEDS

The art of sprouting seeds is as old as recorded history. The use of sprouts was recorded in China as long ago as 2939 B.C. For a millennium, the majority of human foods came from grain seeds. Rice, millet, barley, oats, corn, sorghum, and rye have been staples throughout the globe. Legume seeds are also primary food sources. Lentils, dry beans, dry peas, and soybeans are rich in protein and carbohydrates. Other sources of seed foods are nuts such as almonds and walnuts.

Sprouted seeds have the reputation of power, which they get through the period of germination. Germination is the resumption of growth of a plant seed, spore, or bud after a period of dormancy. The main feature of germination is the increased rate of respiration, which is the biological "burning," or oxidation, of carbohydrate to provide energy for metabolism and growth. The viability, or the ability to germinate after prolonged periods of time, varies greatly among different species. The seeds are potent after they have germinated into sprouts. That is when we eat them. The most popular seeds used for sprouting are alfalfa, mung bean, chick-pea, and lentil.

In the West, sprouts were virtually unheard of a decade or two ago. Today, they are widely used in American cuisine in salads, as a replacement for lettuce on sandwiches, and in Chinese dishes.

YOGURT

Yogurt, a fermented, slightly acidic food product, is made from milk. Its origins are unknown although the name comes from the Turkish language. Yogurt resembles the many other fermented milk foods made throughout the world, such as kefir and kumiss. Unlike many of these foods, however, yogurt is usually made from a concentrated milk and is soured by a specific bacillus, *Lactobacillus bulgaricus.*

During the late nineteenth century, Elie Metchnikoff, a Russian biologist who worked in the Pasteur Institute in Paris, put forward the theory that the deterioration of the body was largely influenced by putrefactive bacteria that produced toxins in the large intestine. Noting the health and longevity of certain Balkan tribes for whom yogurt was a food staple, Metchnikoff suggested that these toxin-producing bacteria could be suppressed by encouraging the growth in the intestine of the lactobacilli from yogurt. His theory was later questioned by bacteriologists who felt that the usual presence of intestinal bile salts might inhibit the proliferation of the "good" bacteria. Nevertheless, many still believe in yogurt's beneficial effects. Additionally, the food has recently become popular as a pleasant, low-calorie alternative to ice cream. The introduction of fruit yogurt during the 1940s revolutionized the market. Until recently, yogurt sales increased by 20 percent or so every year.

Commercial yogurt is made by heating concentrated milk, or milk fortified by skim milk powder, to about 90°C (194°F) for a few minutes, then cooling it to about 44°C (111°F), at which point a controlled culture of *Lactobacillus bulgaricus* and *Streptococcus thermophilus* is added. These two lactic organisms produce the required acidity and the delicate yogurt flavor. Souring and thickening take place in about 3 hours at 44°C (111°F), and stop when the mixture is cooled to 5°C (40°F). Because the milk has been heated and soured, and because of its high acidity, pathogens cannot grow in yogurt. It is probably the safest of all perishable foods. Well-made yogurt of any type should last for 14 days if kept at 5°C (41°F).

Many people make their own yogurt. Yogurt makers can be purchased at most large department stores, and they come with complete instructions for home yogurt preparation. They are available in various cup sizes, usually making six one-to-two cup quantities. When you make yogurt yourself, you are the judge of how much sweetener or natural fruits to add and whether or not to make it with nonfat or whole milk. Of course, you need the culture to begin your first batch, but after that you can start the next lot from an unused container from the previous batch. We make ours with skim milk and add honey and fresh fruits for sweeteners. It stores well in the refrigerator for several days.

SALADS

Growing your own fruits and vegetables can be really wonderful. The joy of gardening is more than just getting to harvest the best and freshest of table treats. The entire process is nourishing. The steps of gardening include preparing the soil, planting the seeds or seedlings, cultivating and weeding the plot, watering and watching the growth, and finally harvesting the fruits or vegetables. What a joy it is to eat your own home-grown tomato or fruit or to toss a green salad from your fresh picked leaves. Not only does the dish taste better, but there is also no doubt that it is packed with more nutrients. None have been lost in the packaging, storage, shipment, and delivery stages that are unfortunately a part of contemporary life. The food goes directly from the harvest to your body. This is the essence of eating living foods. If you have never tried a garden or do not have the space for it, just try a tomato plant or two in pots on your patio. You should be pleased with the process and the results.

SUMMARY

Fresh green salads, yogurt, and seed sprouts are examples of living foods. The more foods are processed, the fewer natural vitamins and minerals remain as the process of cooking and canning tend to deplete vitamin and mineral stores. Living foods offer us an opportunity to ingest vibrant living cells that work to energize our bodies.

13 HEALING HERBS

Among the various sources of nutrition, there are those substances that concentrate chemicals and produce particular salutary effects on our systems. This general category is referred to as herbs. Herbs may be used in small quantities in cooking and food preparation where their aromatic properties add color, flavor, aroma, and zest, as well as in tisanes and teas where they may soothe, stimulate, relax, and console us while providing a contemplative and communicative environment. In high concentrations, they may be used therapeutically.

One caution about herbs is that they can be toxic when misused. Most commercial preparations are completely safe. However, when formulating your own teas and compounds, refer to at least three different reference sources to validate the safety of your recipe. Some common herbs, such as angelica and sassafras, can be carcinogenic. Other commonly used herbs, such as saffron, can be, in high concentrations, toxic to the heart and liver. Foxglove, from which digitalis was originally made, can in very minute dosages stimulate the heart, but in slightly higher doses, it can produce cardiac arrhythmias and has been incriminated in numerous fatalities. On the other hand, with the proper knowledge, herbs can serve both as supplements for healing and in the prevention of illness and disease.

This chapter serves as a cursory introduction to the use of herbs. If you would like to pursue this fascinating art, you will probably want to collect individual herb books and begin experimental cultivation of your own small herb garden.

THE SALUTARY EFFECTS OF HERBS

Studying, cultivating, and using herbs can be a transformative process. As you work with herbs, you become more deeply involved with the natural processes and interactions of the healing substances of the earth. You experience the rewards of seeing an organism that you plant and nurture with your own hands transformed by the process of nature. With daily involvement, you become part of birth, dying, rebirth, and transmutation.

Herbalism becomes a holistic process encompassing not only physiological body effects, but those involving the mind, emotions, and spirit. Herbs can be another effective dietary tool when used properly as supplements to food. They aid in the prevention of disease through their ability to modulate and strengthen the immune system.

SOURCES OF HERBS

The best sources of herbs are those that you grow or gather and prepare yourself. This enables you to participate entirely in the process of birth, growth, and transformation of the substance. As you grow or gather herbs, you have the opportunity to experience the true essence of the substance and benefit in multiple ways from the use of it. When herbs are purchased from commercial sources, they should be used in some symbolic way in order to obtain maximum benefit on each level of the body-mind-spirit template.

Growing your own herbs gives you complete control over the environment in which they are grown. You control the soil content, quantity of water, and nutrients, as well as share in the aesthetic process of growth, fruition, and harvest.

When gathering wild herbs, you must know herbs well and harvest far from roads and sources of pollution. Herbs gathered too close to roads will have high concentrations of lead, arsenicals, and other toxins. Some people, such as the Tibetan monks of the high Himalayas, think only wild herbs are useful. Most of us, however, live in a much different environment. Consequently, we must alter our opinions of what is useful.

With the exception of standard teas, when purchasing commercial preparations, it is essential to examine the herb, cross-reference it in an herb book or manual, and use only small quantities until the potency of the preparation can be ascertained.

PREPARATION OF HERBS FOR USE

Several terms are important in understanding the preparation of herbs.

Infusion An infusion or a tisane is a fancy name for a tea. You can use either fresh (preferably) or dried leaves of the herb (generally 3 parts fresh is the equivalent of 1 part dried). Place them into a well-warmed teapot and add about 1 cup of boiling water per 3 teaspoons dried herbs. Then steep the mixture for 10 to 15 minutes. Sweeten the mixture with licorice root, honey, or sugar to make it more palatable. Use infusions immediately; do not store them.

Crushing or grinding the leaves and seeds may enhance the extraction of the volatile oils. You may prefer cold infusions of herbs with highly volatile oils. This is accomplished by placing the herb in a sealed glass container and steeping for a period of 12 hours.

One of my favorite sources for obtaining medicinal teas is Traditional Medicinal, Inc., 4515 Ross Road, Sebastopol, CA 95472. These teas are excellent preparations which are effective, easily prepared, and require minimal effort.

Decoction When the herb used is a hard or woody stem, root, or bark such as willow or a hard seed or nut, it is better to use a decoction as opposed to an infusion. The proportions of fresh or dried herbs are the same as with an infusion—3 teaspoons of fresh herb or 1 teaspoon of dried to 1 cup of water. However, after breaking the herb into small pieces, you should simmer it in water in a covered pot for varying periods of time, depending on which herb you are using, and then strain the solution. It is important to use glass vessels rather than metal (especially aluminum) vessels because the boiling of the decoction could extract harmful substances from the metal. The importance of avoiding aluminum cookware in general cannot be overemphasized. The decoction can be refrigerated, but it is best used immediately.

Tinctures   A tincture is a solution of the herb in an alcohol base. Alcohol is a better solvent and preservative for most plant derivatives than water. Alcohol derivatives of herbs are called tinctures. Preparations can also be made from vinegar and glycerine.

The easiest way to make a tincture is to use vodka or brandy. Place 2 ounces of dried herbs or 4 ounces of fresh herbs in a sealed glass container with 1 cup of vodka or brandy and set the container in a warm place. Shake it periodically. Allow the mixture to steep for 2 to 4 hours and then filter it through a cheesecloth. Tinctures are quite stable and may last for years. You can make tinctures with wine, but they will have a shorter shelf life. For example, Rosemary wine can be used as an effective digestive herb.

Tinctures are much stronger than infusions or decoctions. The dosage, therefore, is smaller. Generally, 5 to 15 drops added to hot or cold sweetened water is the best method of using the tincture. Creative herbalists can create their own tarragon, rosemary, or basil vinegars using these herbs in apple cider vinegar.

Syrups for coughs can be made using the appropriate herbs dissolved in a syrup made from a 2-to-3 dilution of sugar and water. The tincture is then added to the sugar syrup in a 1-part tincture to 3-part syrup mixture.

DRYING OF HARVESTED HERBS

The most expedient method of drying grown or gathered herbs is to use a commercially obtained dehydrator. The temperature should be set low, about 95 to 100°F.

A more aesthetic and personal way to dehydrate herbs is by using an ordinary lunch-sack-size, brown paper bag. Prepare the bag by turning down the top to form a cuff. Make several down rolls until the bag is about two-thirds open. Place the herbs in the base of the bag and put it in a warm location, such as on top of the refrigerator. This location allows you to subconsciously notice its presence, which is nice since it reminds you that you are personally involved in the whole process of the preparation. As your herbs dry, the aromas will permeate the surrounding environment. Another method you may want to try is to bundle, tie into a bunch, and hang your herbs from the ceiling or doorway frame. In addition to enjoying the aroma, you will have the aesthetic pleasure of seeing your herbs swaying in the breeze.

Herbs are best stored in airtight, sealed containers. The best containers are corked brown jars. Store the containers in a cool, dark place. For convenience, I store my herbs in ziplock freezer bags in a cool, dark, dry environment.

HERBAL CONSTITUENTS

The substances within herbs are the products and gifts of a fruitful and loving earth. They sustain us by a process of synergism; that is, multiple substances interacting with one another.

Numerous substances, including water, organic and inorganic compounds, sugars, and carbohydrates, are present in herbs. Weak acids are present in herbs such as cranberries. These acids may be useful in the prevention and treatment of urinary tract infections. The "sting" of the nettle plant is related to a weak organic acid.

Some herbs contain alcohol substances. Alcohols such as the menthol in peppermint may be useful in the treatment of respiratory and congestive problems.

Most herbs contain multiple volatile oils which delight our senses, stimulate us, and have therapeutic value. Think of the odors of peppermint, thyme, rosemary, eucalyptus, and garlic. Such oils have both local and systemic effects. After we ingest them, they diffuse to many systems throughout our bodies.

Some of the herbal oils have been found to strengthen our immune systems by a process of "immune modulation." When the herbal substance combines with our internal knowledge systems, it seems to provide our bodies with whatever substance they need, having different effects in different individuals. The effects are modulated not only through our organ systems themselves, but also centrally where the taste and odor of the oil stimulates the olfactory system. This system, which is directly connected with the brain, stimulates feelings of inner peace and well-being, which further modulates the immune mechanism.

Plant sugars and carbohydrates can serve as energy sources and can be used in the process of fermentation. Herbs such as grapes can be made into wines which "gladden" the heart and may produce (in proper quantities) beneficial effects on the cardiac and immune systems.

Phenolic compounds (chemical structures) such as the derivative of willow bark (acetylsalicylic acid or aspirin) and the oil of cloves and thyme are painkillers. The salutary effects of barberry on the urinary tract may be explained by the phenolic compounds. Indeed, a whole new class of antibiotics named the "quinolones" has been based on similar compounds.

Numerous other substances such as tannins, coumanins, glycosides, saponins, and alkaloids are all found in plant substances and interact with one another. Proper and full knowledge of these substances is leading to more incredible medical discoveries each day. For example, digitalis is a cardiac glycoside and coumanins are anticoagulants. When used in small dosages, the effects of these substances can prevent disease and stimulate all our organ systems.

POPULAR HERBS

The following herbs are readily available, either self-grown or obtained at the local health food market.

Aloe   Aloe is easily grown and is best used externally for insect bites, sunburn, and minor burns. It can be used internally as a cathartic, but I do not recommend this.

Aniseed   This can be used as a delicious mystery seasoning in bouillabaisse and seafood dishes. Used medicinally in combination with other herbs, it is effective in respiratory problems and is calming to the bowel.

Balm or lemon balm This can be used in salads, but the most delicious teas are produced from the fresh or dried leaves. I can attest that it has definite calming effects on tensions after a hard day's work. It reduces stress, lightens depression and anxiety, and is effective for digestive disorders. It can be used to supplement lemon verbena and can be combined with most other herbs.

Basil Basil can be easily obtained as an annual from most nurseries and adds a delightful touch to salads. My favorite use for it is as a key ingredient in making pesto sauce for fettuccine.

Bearberry Combined with easily gathered yarrow, bearberry can be used as a supplementary treatment for urinary disorders, including gravel (small kidney stones) in the urinary tract.

Borage The use of borage as a tea made from dried leaves is reputed to be a restorative to the adrenal glands and, as such, is said to be effective in chronic stress syndromes. I use the flowers as decorations on salads and the finely chopped leaves directly in the salad. The flavor is somewhat like cucumber with slightly fishy overtones. Consequently, this pungent herb may not be appreciated by everyone. One of its assets is that it is easily grown.

Caraway Caraway is readily available as seeds, which should be crushed to make tea. It is reputed to be effective for flatulence and colic, and when combined with other agents, it may be effective for bronchitis. For zest and texture, add it to your homemade breads. Caraway is the flavorful ingredient in the Scandinavian drink, Aqua Vita.

Cardomon These seeds are grown on the Indian subcontinent and provide an interesting effect when used in breads or added to beverages. They can be used medicinally as an appetite stimulant and as a treatment for dyspepsia. This herb is very effective when used for respiratory conditions.

Cascara Made from treebark, cascara can be used as a mild purgative.

Chamomile These flowers can be combined in teas to aid in digestion.

Cinnamon   Made from treebark, cinnamon is a common culinary herb that can also be used to relieve nausea and vomiting and stabilize the bowel.

Cloves   Cloves are similar in effect to cinnamon. They may also be useful for toothaches.

Coriander   These seeds are used in pickling spices and, especially when ground, add unique flavor to rice dishes. A coriander rice dish is beneficial to the bowel.

Cucumber   Cucumber is delicious in salads. The topical application of cucumber juice soothes and cools the skin. Preparations made from cucumber are used in salons for facials.

Cumin   Similar to coriander, cumin adds warmth to soups and stews, and is an ingredient in curry.

Damiana   Tea made with damiana can be used for anxiety and depression. It is said to be a male sexual stimulant.

Dandelion   Dandelion leaves are good in salads. Less commonly used, but equally edible, are the prepared roots. Dandelion can be used medicinally as a powerful diuretic.

Dill   Dill weed and seeds can be used in salads. The tea can be used as a remedy for flatulence.

Eichenacea   This is said to be a good immune system stimulant. The decoction of the root may be helpful in laryngitis and cystitis.

Ephedra   Commercially known as MaHuang, ephedra is quite clearly of benefit in asthmatic conditions, as well as allergic problems such as hayfever.

Fennel   Delicious in salads, fennel is quite flavorful. An infusion of the crushed seeds is helpful in relieving colic and flatulence.

Fenugreek seeds   These seeds are an ancient remedy for localized wounds. The seeds make an interesting tea with a slight hint of curry. The sprouts are exotic when used in salads.

Garlic Garlic is the universal adaptogen that aids us in many ways. It has antibacterial, antiviral, and antiparasitic properties. It is said to help prevent heart disease and cancer; lower blood pressure and cholesterol levels; and it can be used with other herbs in the treatment of bronchitis and asthma.

Ginger The roots can be used to produce diaphoresis and to aid digestion.

Gentian Used either as a tincture or a decoction, this root is said to be an appetite stimulant.

Ginseng The roots have been firmly established in the medical literature as an adaptogen. The regular use of ginseng as an infusion or decoction is said to be an antidepressant and improves physical and mental performance.

Hawthorne When used in the proper mixture and proportions, these berries have been found to reduce blood pressure.

Hops The hops flowers are an excellent treatment for insomnia, especially when combined with Valerian. The shelf life for the flowers is quite limited.

Horseradish Horseradish makes an excellent sauce when ground. It can be used as an infusion that is helpful in influenza and fevers as well as in bronchitis.

Horsetail This is commonly available along paths and roads. The dried stems and leaves can be made into an infusion that is helpful in the treatment of prostate problems. When combined with saw palmetto berries, it may actually be able to shrink enlarged prostates. However, the scientific information about this use is scant.

Juniper The berries add an interesting flavor to wild game and to rice and wheat pilafs. The infusion is said to be helpful in rheumatism and cystitis, but should be avoided in kidney disease. Medically, it should be used with caution.

Lavender Lavender is delightful to the eye and has a lovely aroma. The flowers and leaves are used in potpourris. The oil can be rubbed on the skin, but avoid any internal use, even in salads.

Licorice   Made from the glycerrhiza root (meaning sweet root), licorice can be used as the basis of many infusions and delightful teas. When combined with other herbs, it is effective as a treatment for bronchitis. It also has salutary effects on the gastrointestinal system. Its overuse, however, should be avoided by persons with high blood pressure.

Marjoram   Easily grown, marjoram makes an excellent addition to stews, salads, and soups. Infusions from marjoram may be useful for headaches.

Mullein   The flower is steeped in hot water until the water is yellow. The tea relieves persistent cough, respiratory mucus, and hoarseness.

Mustard   The seeds, when crushed in warm water, are used to induce vomiting. Mustard is used in powdered form to make a poultice that draws blood to the skin and relieves pain and inflammation in rheumatism and arthritis.

These are but a few of the healing herbs. Many others such as nasturtium, nettles, oats, parsley, peppermint, pumpkin, raspberry, red clover, red sage, rose hips, rosemary, saw palmetto, thyme, valerian, and yarrow all have healing medicinal uses.

SUMMARY

Studying, cultivating, and using herbs can contribute to personal empowerment. Herbalism can be a holistic process engaging all our physical senses while at the same time involving our minds and spirits. Herbs, used in the proper doses and mixtures, can be among the most healing of all our foods.

Suggested Reading

Bremness, L. (1988). *The complete book of herbs.* New York: Viking Studio Books.

Hoffman, D. (1992). *The new holistic herbal.* Rockport, MA: Element, Inc.

Kadans, J. (1970). *Encyclopedia of medicinal herbs.* New York: Arco Publishing, Inc.

Kowalchik, C., & Hylton, W. (Eds.). (1987). *Rodales' illustrated encyclopedia of herbs.* Emmaus, PA: Rodale Press.

Lust, J. (1974). *The herb book.* New York: Bantam Books.

Mabey, R. (Ed.). (1988). *The new age herbalist.* New York: Collier Books.

Thomas, L. (1990). *10 essential herbs.* Prescott, AZ: Hahn Press.

Tierra, M. (1980). *The way of herbs.* New York: Washington Square Press.

Weiss, G., & Weiss, S. (1985). *Growing and using the healing herbs.* Emmaus, PA: The Rodale Press.

14 VEGETARIANISM

People who abstain from foods of animal origin are vegetarians. The first of several subcategories include those who refer to themselves as vegans and avoid all animal foods. The second group, the lacto-ovo-vegetarians, allow eggs and dairy products in their diets. Because egg whites and some dairy products are outstanding protein sources and fair sources of vitamin B_{12}, the lacto-ovo-vegetarian diet can easily be a nutritious one. A true vegan diet, without eggs and dairy products, takes greater attention, planning, and knowledge to maintain adequate intake and optimal health. Unbalanced vegetarian diets can result in scurvy, anemia, protein starvation, and death. A third variation of the vegetarian diet is the macrobiotic diet, which includes whole grains, legumes, vegetables, and other staples of the Eastern world. Technically, macrobiotic followers may not be true vegetarians since some fish and seafood products may be included.

The newest addition to these terms is *vegetarian awareness*. This term indicates a necessary awareness by all of us who deal with foods. We all probably know people who are vegetarians. If we do not understand this dietary variation, we probably wonder about the adequacy of their diet, the reasons for their variation, and why and how they eat in this way.

HISTORY

Although this mode of nutrition has had a limited historical practice in North America, it has been followed for centuries in places such as the Asian subcontinent. However, vegetarianism is not historically restricted to the East. The sixth century Greek philosopher Pythagoras and others abstained from meat eating based primarily on their beliefs in the transmigration of souls. In the eighteenth century, Benjamin Franklin in America and Voltaire in France were prominent advocates of vegetarianism. Although there have always been members of this sect, the rapid growth of this movement in the United States has occurred chiefly during the past two decades. Today there are millions of practicing vegetarians, with books, journals, seminars, and meetings to aid and abet them in the pursuit of clean, wholesome, healthful eating.

WHY BE A VEGETARIAN?

There are several reasons why people subscribe to vegetarianism. Perhaps the primary one is related to religious beliefs. In religions that affirm a belief in reincarnation, a multilife kinship between humans and animals, the eating of flesh is forbidden. The belief is that if you do not surmount certain problems in this life, then it is possible to be born again in the lower lifeform of an animal. Since you would not want to take the chance of consuming a friend or relative, or having your heirs consume you, then eating of all animal flesh is taboo.

A second reason people adhere to a diet devoid of meat relates to their environmental concerns. People concerned about the ability of the planet to produce sufficient quantities of food to sustain a burgeoning population think that reducing meat consumption will help. For example, an acre of land will yield a much greater quantity of edible plant food than animal meat (see "Soybeans" later in this chapter, and "Sprouts" in chapter 12 for additional information). An acre of land can produce as much as 385 pounds of alfalfa seed from 1 pound of seed. If 384 pounds were sprouted for food, the yield would be approximately 3,180 pounds of consumable sprouts. Thus, we can see why consumption of protein-containing sprouted food could make a significant environmental difference.

A third reason for vegetarianism relates to health. Many advocates of this lifestyle are queasy about the sanitation of production houses, slaughter methods, and possible contamination of the meat itself during the transportation, storage, and preparation process.

In the United States, approximately 1 million farmers and ranchers raise livestock, which is slaughtered at approximately 6,000 federally inspected plants, which do more than 97 percent of all processing. Currently, four major packers process approximately 70 percent of the beef and another four about 60 percent of the pork in the United States. Although The Humane Slaughter Act (1960) requires that prior to slaughter animals be rendered completely unconscious with a minimum of excitement and discomfort using mechanical, electrical, or chemical (carbon dioxide gas) methods, some people contend that this practice is not followed as closely as it should be.

The Seventh-Day Adventist (SDA) religious community comprises an enormous group of vegetarians worldwide. To support their tenets on the health benefits of this lifestyle, they continually collect data to demonstrate its benefits. They contend that

- SDA men 55 and over who eat meat 6 or more times a week are twice as likely to die of heart disease as vegetarian SDAs.

- SDA men aged 40 to 54 who eat meat 6 or more times a week have 4 times the risk of a fatal heart attack than do vegetarian SDAs.

- SDA meat-eating women over 55 have 1.5 times the risk of a fatal heart attack than do female vegetarian SDAs.

Even the conservative American Dietetic Association recognizes that a growing body of scientific evidence supports a positive relationship between the consumption of a plant-based diet and the prevention of certain diseases. The meat industry denies the health benefits of vegetarian diets, but research on cancer, heart disease, high blood pressure, diabetes, and obesity might lead us to argue otherwise. The average blood cholesterol level of vegetarians is about 125, which is much lower than that of average Americans. Because they eat less fat and more grains, legumes, and vegetables, vegetarians appear to be healthier than average Americans.

ADEQUACY OF NUTRIENTS IN THE DIET

It is quite possible for vegetarians to obtain all the nutrients they need. Studies conducted at the University of Belgium at the beginning of this century compared endurance, strength, and quickness of recovery from fatigue in vegetarians and meat eaters. The findings indicated that vegetarians were superior in all three characteristics. Replicated studies in 1907 at Yale University and in 1909 at Battle Creek Sanitarium in Michigan confirmed the original findings.

Lacto-ovo-vegetarians gained international recognition in 1917–1918 during World War I when a group of captive Danes were deprived of meat and forced to subsist on grains, fruits, and dairy products. To the great surprise of their captors, they exhibited improved health and lowered death rates.

Amino Acids

In the early 1900s chemical analysis of foods began to provide a scientific basis for nutrition. The essential amino acids were determined, vitamins were isolated, and minerals were identified. Protein is an essential element in the diet. The amino acid building blocks must be available to the cytoplasm. Many amino acids are synthesized in our bodies, but some are not. Those not synthesized are called essential. They include isoleucine, leucine, lysine, methionine, phenylalanine, threonine, tryptophan, and valine. These amino acids must be provided in the foods we eat.

One of the potential problems in vegetarianism is that nearly all types of vegetable protein are deficient in certain essential amino acids. The notable exception is soybeans. That is why this food is one of the essential ingredients in the vegan's diet. In addition to using soybeans, certain foods can be combined throughout the day to create complete proteins. For example, eating corn and beans, rice and beans, or coupling certain cereals with legumes produces a complete protein.

Knowing this information helps health professionals to teach good vegetarian eating combinations. In the southern United States and Mexico, for example, corn is a staple. If people ate corn alone, their diets would be deficient in tryptophan and lysine, and their growth and tissue replacement would be impaired. By combining corn with eggs, milk, or beans, vegans can balance their diets. Vegetarian peoples of interior Africa and India tend to suffer from protein deficiencies that their coastal brothers and sisters avoid because coastal residents supplement their diets with fish. In these areas, there is a significant need for nutritional teaching utilizing locally available foods.

One possible hazard of the vegan diet is an extreme reduction in saturated fat and cholesterol intake. Our bodies do produce their own cholesterol when it is not ingested; but we require a certain level of fat intake to maintain homeostasis. The up side of this issue is that vegetarians may have a lower risk for coronary artery disease since they do not have the saturated fat intake to build up atherosclerotic plaques along their vessel walls.

ADVANTAGES AND DISADVANTAGES OF VEGETARIAN DIETS

Advantages

While there may be some disadvantages to a vegetarian diet, there are specific advantages. These include:

- Increased fiber. Vegetables and fruits are high in fiber compared to fleshy meat. Increased fiber aids in bowel movements and helps to prevent problems such as diverticulitis and colon cancer.

- Decreased daily caloric intake. Vegetables tend to be low in calories, so a vegetarian diet is beneficial to people trying to maintain or lose weight.

- Decreased total fat, saturated fat, and cholesterol intake. Since fruits and vegetables are low in fat and cholesterol compared to meat, vegetarian diets can be beneficial to people with hyperlipidemia (elevated level of lipids in the blood) and can decrease the risk of developing atherosclerosis.

- Financial economy. Meat is often expensive. A vegetarian diet provides an affordable source of protein.

Possible Disadvantages

- Protein deficiency. See the section in this chapter on combining grains and legumes, for example.

- Flatulence. When you begin a vegetarian diet, the bowel needs time to adjust to the increased amount of fiber. Until the bowel adjusts to a slower rate, frequent bowel movements and flatus may occur. However, new products are available that can be added in small amounts to food servings. These derivatives of molds can aid in digestion, thus decreasing flatulence. If you are allergic to medicines such as penicillin, however, you should probably avoid these products because you might be allergic to the antigas formula as well. One commercially available product for this condition is "Beano™."

WHAT TO EAT

Most new vegans quickly learn the proper balance of whole grains, vegetables, fruits, legumes, nuts, and seeds. These people generally do not waste any part of their daily caloric intake on empty calories such as candy, cakes, sodas, or other foods that have no nutritional value.

The Macrobiotic Diet

Macrobiotics refers to a way of eating based on choosing and preparing foods in harmony with nature and in accordance with our individual needs. By promoting a diet low in fat, high in complex carbohydrates and fiber, and nearly cholesterolfree, macrobiotics promotes the concept of the link between healthy diet and healthy lifestyle.

In the macrobiotic diet, all foods are categorized as either being yin (expansive, relaxing, or diffusive) or yang (contractive or having a focused effect). Meat and salt, for example, are highly contractive yang foods. In a meal containing these foods, more expansive yin foods such as vegetables should be eaten to bring the contractive foods into balance. Advocates of this regimen believe that an excessive yang diet can result in overly contractive physical or emotional tendencies, such as hypertension or feeling "uptight." At the opposite extreme, an overly yin diet can make us feel unmotivated or uncoordinated physically and emotionally. The goal in macrobiotics is to avoid either extreme and to eat foods that are more balanced within themselves and to one another. Within this system, food should also be balanced with activity level and the weather. For example, on a cold day, you drink warm teas to balance the temperature. Even illnesses are categorized as yin or yang and are balanced accordingly with proper food and treatment.

Those who eat from a macrobiotic source seek food in its most natural state: fresh, locally grown when possible, grown without chemical fertilizers or pesticides, and free of additives and preservatives. Dairy products and highly refined carbohydrates are discouraged.

The standard macrobiotic diet usually consists of 50 percent grains, 25 percent vegetables, 5 to 10 percent beans and sea vegetables, 5 percent soup, and 5 percent condiments and other foods. Whole grains, including brown rice, millet, barley, oats, buckwheat, quinoa, rye, amaranth, corn, and whole wheat are cooked with sea salt to enhance digestibility. For optimum nutrition, whole grains are preferable to white breads and noodles.

Depending on the climate, season, and our individual needs, it is suggested that at least two-thirds of the vegetables be steamed, boiled, baked, or sauteed, while one-third may be eaten raw. Persons living in temperate zones should consume vegetables and fruits grown in a similar climate or, preferably, the same region. Nonindigenous foods such as bananas, pineapple, and even potatoes and tomatoes are not recommended for frequent use.

Sea vegetables are especially high in minerals such as calcium. They can be cooked with beans, soups, and vegetables or made into side dishes cooked and seasoned with soy sauce.

Soup made with fermented soybean paste called miso (pronounced "mee-so") is generally eaten on a daily basis. Unpasteurized miso is abundant in lactobacillus bacteria and enzymes, which reportedly aid digestion and food assimilation. Miso should be added to soup stock at the end of cooking and should not be boiled. This preserves the "good" bacteria and the enzymes.

Condiments, especially sesame salt (commonly known as gomasio; pronounced "go-mah-see-o"), are used to enhance flavor, add nutrition, promote better digestion, and help balance the meal with regard to the yin and yang. Traditional pickles such as daikon radish, sauerkraut, and rice bran pickles are an important part of this whole grain-based diet.

Twig tea, barley tea, grain coffees, and noncarbonated mineral water are the beverages of choice in the macrobiotic diet.

Soybeans

Soybeans are one of the most important sources of protein known to humankind. Soybean crops can produce over 33 percent more protein from an acre of land than any other known crop and 20 times as much usable protein as can be raised on an acre of land used for grazing cattle. The yield of protein is high, both in terms of quantity and quality. Soybeans contain about 35 percent protein, more than any other unprocessed plant or animal food. Another exceptional quality of soy protein is that it includes all of the eight essential amino acids in a configuration readily usable by the human body. For example, a 1/2-cup serving of usable soy protein is equivalent to 5 ounces of steak. The difference between the two is that the soybeans have no cholesterol or saturated fats.

The United States now produces about two-thirds of the world's soybeans. Actually, soybeans are one of our largest crops, second only to corn and wheat. There is enough grown each year to provide every American with their full RDA requirements for three years. If the soybeans produced in the United States were distributed equally among all the people on the planet, they would fulfill about 25 percent of their yearly protein requirements. However, the vast majority of these soybeans never reach human beings. They are exported, extracted for oil, or used as feed for livestock.

Almost all of America's nonexported soybeans go to factories where millions of pounds a day are converted to soy oil. This oil, which contains no protein, is refined and sold as cooking or salad oil. Defatted soybean meal is the primary by-product of the oil extraction process. This meal contains about 2 1/2 times as much protein by weight as steak. What happens to the meal? It is fed to livestock. In addition to this prize protein, we feed livestock 78 percent of all our grain. Both the soybeans and the grain could be used directly as food for people. As a society, we have yet to understand and utilize soybeans as an important food source.

The soybeans utilized for human consumption are hallmarks of many vegetarian diets. The foods derived from soybeans are tofu, miso (fermented soybean paste), and shoyu (natural soy sauce). Miso is often served as a soup and shoyu is used as a high-protein seasoning. Tofu is used as the backbone of the vegetarian diet in much the same way as meat and dairy products are used in the typical American diet.

Tofu is a colorless bean curd that comes in a variety of shapes and forms and can be cut, fried, baked, or ground to use in any cooking combination. It is prepared by a process that removes the crude fiber, making it much easier to digest than the meats and grains we ordinarily eat. Babies, the elderly, and people with digestive problems can thrive on tofu.

Tofu is low in calories. An 8-ounce serving of eggs has about 450 calories. An 8-ounce serving of meat has about 600 calories, while the same amount of tofu contains only 150 calories. We know there is a correlation between overweight and consumption of large amounts of animal foods high in saturated fats. Research studies show that American vegetarians are 20 pounds below the national average. In countries with relatively low meat consumption, such as Japan and India, the people are close to their ideal body weights.

We know that herbicides, pesticides, and heavy metals tend to concentrate in the fatty tissues of animals at the top of the food chain. Fish, poultry, and meat contain about 20 times more pesticide residues than legumes. Because soybeans are a legume crop at the base of the food chain, their spraying is carefully monitored by the Food and Drug Administration to keep the level of contamination at a minimum. Soybean foods in the diet have been found to lower the risk of breast cancer in pre-menopausal women (Cassidy, Bingham, & Setchell, in press). In general, soy products have been found to be helpful in preventing colon, prostate, and breast cancer (Messina & Barnes, 1991).

There are many reasons to use tofu in our diets. Tofu is

- an excellent source of calcium—an 8-ounce serving provides 38 percent RDA of calcium.

- an excellent source of iron, phosphorus, potassium, sodium, essential B vitamins, choline, and fat-soluble vitamin E.

- a high-quality protein.

- easy to digest.

- low in saturated fats and cholesterol.

- free of chemical toxins.

- helpful for preventing cancer.

- low in cost.

- versatile and easy to use.

Buying and Using Tofu

Most grocery stores now carry tofu. It is often found in the fresh produce section or in the refrigerator section near the dairy products. Fresh packaged tofu comes in a plastic container with a date stamped on the outside. Buy the product with the most recent date. If an expiration date has been reached, do not buy the product. Ask the produce manager to get fresh stock from the storeroom. If none is available postpone your purchase of tofu.

After you bring your fresh tofu home from the store, keep it under constant refrigeration until you are ready to use it. If you must postpone preparing your tofu dish for several days, you can store it by slitting the top of the plastic seal, draining the water contents, and refilling the package around the tofu with new water. You can drain and refill for up to ten days without product spoilage. There will be some loss of texture and flavor, but the nutrient value will remain intact.

Once you begin cooking with tofu, you will awaken to a world of recipes and uses for this versatile food. You will discover dishes that can be enjoyed from breakfast to dinners to desserts. With tofu, you can create sauces, soups, toppings, dressings, stocks, and entrées. Table 14.1 gives you a few ideas.

Breakfast

Butter-fried tofu
Scrambled tofu eggs
Pan-fried tofu
Tofu fruit whips

Lunch and Dinner Dishes

Tofu spaghetti sauce
Tofu cottage cheese
Carrot and raisin salad with tofu
Tofu guacamole
Tofu burgers
Curried rice with tofu
Crisp deep-fried tofu
Chunky tofu and pineapple

Desserts

Fresh fruit salad with tofu whipped cream
Tofu peanut butter and banana spread
Tofu cheesecake
Tofu pudding

TABLE 14.1   Tofu Meal Ideas

SUMMARY

Vegetarianism is experiencing a renaissance in the American diet. Increasing numbers of people are eating meatless diets and seeming to thrive while doing so. In order to follow and benefit from this dietary regime, it is important to understand how to select and prepare meals to ensure proper intake of all the essential nutrients.

References

Cassidy, A., Bingham, S., & Setchell, K. D. (in press). Biological effects of isoflavones present in soy in premenopausal women: Implications for the prevention of breast cancer. *American Journal of Clinical Nutrition.*

Messina, M. J., & Barnes, S. (1991). The role of soy products in reducing the risk of cancer. *Journal of the National Cancer Institute, 83,* 541–546.

15 | THE JOYS OF JUICING

WHAT IS JUICING?

Juicing is drinking fresh raw juice from fruits and vegetables. The theory of juicing is that by using the freshest fruits and vegetables we can obtain, we will have more energy and increased health and vitality. Proponents believe we will heal faster, build our immune systems, and even look younger. Anyone can juice. It is easy, quick, and may even save us money because we will eat fewer high-priced, commercially prepared, high-calorie, high-fat meals.

HOW JUICING WORKS

Within the fiber cells of every fresh fruit and vegetable are the liquids that contain the life-sustaining elements that nature provides. These elements are the carbohydrates, protein, fat, minerals, vitamins, bioflavonoids, chlorophyll, and enzymes that we need to nourish our bodies. Juice proponents contend that these life liquids lie in the most difficult part of the plant to reach, locked in the fiber of the plant, the part we call roughage. To get the full benefit of the liquids, some nutritionists think that we need to separate the liquids from the fiber. Until recently, the only way we could access these liquids was by mechanically chewing the raw vegetable or fruit.

Squeezing fruits with a hand-held tool is an alternative to eating the fruit raw, but this leaves much of the vital liquid locked in the peel. It is just not practical to hand squeeze most fruits, let alone vegetables. The alternative to chewing and squeezing is to juice the fruits and vegetables with an electric juicer. Juicing provides us with the full nutritional value of the fruits and vegetables by the masticating action of the juicer, which crushes the fibers and releases the vital liquids from the cells. The drink is pure nutritional power that can be absorbed in our bloodstreams and assimilated in every one of our 60 trillion cells within 15 minutes.

When we drink fresh vegetable and fruit juices, we are giving our bodies instant nutrition. We can feel the effects moments after consuming freshly juiced vegetables and fruits. When we eat the vegetables and fruits raw, our bodies go through a very exhaustive process to extract the juice from the fiber. It is energy consuming, and it takes hours to reap these benefits. Juicing fruits and vegetables is not only a very time-efficient way of getting these life liquids into our bodies, but juicing is also a very effective means of taking in large amounts of carbohydrates, minerals, vitamins, bioflavonoids, chlorophyll, and enzymes. Although we cannot eat 40 carrots or 20 apples or 12 celery stalks a day, we can juice them and consume the fruits and vegetables in a drink. This is an important aspect in the phenomenon of juicing.

Fresh fruits and vegetables are filled with nutrients and enzymes. These enzymes make the nutritional products more available to the cells by speeding their absorption. It is impossible to eat pounds and pounds of raw fruit and vegetables. For one thing, we do not have the time. For another, our systems cannot handle the roughage that would result. We do need roughage in our diets, but too much overburdens our digestive tracts. For example, how long would it take you to eat 1 pound of carrots? Probably quite a while, and it would be even longer until the nutrients were digested, absorbed, and assimilated into your body. Yet 1 pound of carrots can be juiced into one 8-ounce glass of carrot juice that we can drink in a minute. In that one glass there is enough beta carotene to give us 20,000 to 25,000 IU of vitamin A. The RDA minimal requirement is 5,000 units. It also contains potassium, sodium, iron, phosphorous and carbohydrates.

Remember, current recommendations are for meeting minimum daily requirements, or whatever we need to maintain borderline health. However, many nutritionists have begun to reorient their thinking to suggest optimum daily requirements. This means assessing personal daily requirements to represent the balance of vitamins, minerals, and other nutrients we need to maintain our health and lifestyles. To do this, we need to account for individual health problems as well as family history or disease-related illnesses.

Juicing advocates believe that the more fresh, unprocessed foods we eat and the lower on the food chain we eat (meaning more plants), the better our immune systems will function. Eating foods in their natural state, rather than foods that have been processed, canned, or cooked, assures us of receiving the full value of the inherent life-giving substances in those foods. Juicers are quick to point out that we are the only inhabitants on this planet who cook the foods we eat. They contend that cooking severely reduces the nutritional value of foods, leaching away minerals and vitamins by cooking in water, and destroying enzymes through the action of heating.

ENZYMES

A key word for juice advocates is *enzymes*. Actually, enzymes may be the engines of life. Wherever there is life, there are enzymes. Enzymes are like catalysts. They work on a cellular level to promote chemical action without destroying, changing, or using themselves up in the process. They play a role in virtually all body activities. In fact, life could not exist without enzymes despite the presence of sufficient amounts of vitamins, minerals, and water.

Enzymes are sensitive to heat. They begin to be destroyed when exposed to temperatures above 102°F. When the temperature reaches 120°F, they die. Cooked food has no enzymes. Processed foods have no enzymes. Milk and canned juice have no enzymes. When we eat canned fruits and vegetables, we are eating food that has been exposed to high temperatures during the canning process. The government requires those high temperatures to kill bacteria, but unfortunately they also kill enzymes.

Oxygen is one of the most essential elements on earth. As soon as food is cooked, oxygen is lost and enzymes are destroyed. We cannot fully nourish the cells and tissues of our bodies with dead food. The great law of life is replenishment. If we do not eat, we die. If we do not eat the right kinds of foods to nourish our bodies, we may not only die prematurely, but we may suffer along the way.

Our bodies depend upon the quality as well as the quantity of food and its compatibility with the needs of our bodies. We Americans are the best-fed people on the planet, but we are probably the least nutritionally healthy in relation to our wealth. The point here is to begin to believe that we have the power to make ourselves well or ill according to the foods we consume. Unlike medicine, food enables us to build up or tear down the actual tissues of our bodies. When we eat right, we build strong, healthy bodies, but when diets are defective, we tear down our bodies by destroying vital tissue.

Many of us fail to realize that most healing comes from within. Nature has provided us with a wondrous immune system, but we do need to take care of it to enable our internal healing forces to function as they should. Our organs are designed to be self–repairing, but they need the raw materials of life to do their work. Juicing presents that opportunity by delivering the enzyme-rich nourishment of liquids to replenish, repair, and rejuvenate our bodies.

The theory behind fresh, raw vegetable and fruit juices is that they furnish our bodies with the necessary materials for functioning and repair, materials that are so often missing from the average diet. Even if we are not sick, we may not necessarily be healthy. Many people who appear to be in good health have borderline deficiencies, which lead to the eventual breakdown of health and the development of disease. Because of our bodies' miraculous tolerance, months or years may pass before we show any sign of disease.

Many maladies are the result of an incorrect diet. Constipation, folic acid anemia, chronic headaches, nervousness, and stomach trouble respond well to appropriate vegetable juices. The reason is that assimilation of the juices by the body corrects the cell chemistry composition that has become unbalanced through unnatural daily living and dieting habits. Vitality comes from food, and people who lack vitality often have decreased immunity. Deficiency of the primary elements needed in human nutrition is not only the source of most human disease, it is often the origin of mental and spiritual problems as well. People who are not vital lose their love of life.

Raw juice therapy is a natural, drugless therapy soundly advocated by a subset of nutritionists. It is a simple and continuous practice of getting the enzymes of fruits and vegetables inside our systems. It may indeed be the secret to staying young, because with raw juice therapy, we continually revitalize ourselves.

JUICE PREPARATION

If you are interested in the concept of juicing and want to know more, there are recipe books for juices. Juicing recipes tend to fall into two groupings: general daily maintenance juices and specific juices for healing.

An example of a general nutrition juice, which is available in most big-city health food bars, is carrot juice. Gather the ingredients: 5 medium carrots, 1 small apple, 1/2 medium beet.

Wash the carrots and remove their tops. If the apple is waxed, peel it. Remove the core. Scrub and trim the beet. Juice the ingredients and drink.

You may be surprised to learn that there are a number of juice recipes for specific medical conditions. Some of the more general conditions include:

- Acne
- Allergies
- Arthritis
- Asthma
- Backache
- Bladder conditions
- Bronchitis
- Colds
- Constipation
- Dermatitis
- Diarrhea

- Fatigue
- Fever
- Flu
- Gout
- Headache
- Hypertension
- Indigestion
- Insomnia
- Laryngitis
- Sore throat

The key points to remember in preparing juices are:

1. Use the freshest fruits and vegetables that you can obtain. Grow your own if you can. The next best thing is to buy regionally grown products.

2. Buy in season.

3. Wash the produce well.

4. Peel and core fruits, with the exception of grapes and watermelons. You can use the grape peel, but discard the outer watermelon rind.

INTAKE PRINCIPLES

Juice experts advocate following four basic principles for the best use of this method:

1. When you combine two or more products, you change the chemical combination of each one so that the effect of the combination as a whole is different than taking the products individually.

2. Do not mix fruit juices with vegetable juices. The enzymes are not compatible and may cause gastritis. The exception to this principle is apple juice, which generally mixes well with other products.

3. Although you may warm your juice, do not heat it above 130°F or you will destroy the enzymes.

4. When you are ready to drink the juice, take the first mouthful slowly. In order to stimulate the salivary glands to further break down the carbohydrates, you will want to swirl the juice around in your mouth to prepare your digestive system.

I have found that sipping juices over a period of time seems more enjoyable, as well as being easier on the stomach. Remember, this is concentrated food, and your stomach will know it.

SUMMARY

Juicing is a method of vitamin, mineral, and enzyme intake that involves pulverizing fruits and vegetables into a liquid. Fiber is removed and discarded and the remaining liquid is drunk as a meal. Juice is a concentrated food that many advocate for whole body healing.

Suggested Reading

Airola, P. (1991). *Juice fasting.* Sherwood, OR: Health Plus Publishers.

Juicing for health, Audio Seminar (1992). Redmond, WA: Zygon International.

Keane, M. (1992). *Juicing for good health.* New York: Simon & Schuster.

Kirschner, H. E. (1957). *Live food juices.* Monrovia, CA: H.E. Kirschner Publications.

Walker, N. W. (1970). *Fresh vegetable and fruit juices.* Prescott, AZ: Norwalk Press.

16 | THE HEALING POWERS OF WINE

The range and power of modern pharmaceutical agents have given healers new resources to treat infections, soothe chronic pain, and prevent infectious diseases. Yet, despite these technological advances, wine remains one of the safest, easiest to make, and one of the most restorative natural substances on Earth.

Wine differs from most other medicinal agents in that it can also be regarded as a food. It meets the two basic dietary requirements: it provides energy, and it contributes to the maintenance of the body.

When we begin to use wine as a healing food, we can draw with some degree of comfort on intelligent observation and experience recorded over a period of several thousands of years. In addition, we can buttress that lengthy experience with a substantial volume of modern scientific investigation.

WINE USED SENSIBLY

Before addressing the beneficial and medicinal uses of wine, let me first say that it is imperative that this substance be used in moderation and with good judgment. As we all know, there are those who cannot control their intake of alcoholic drinks. Whether this is a genetic trait or a learned behavior is debatable, but the facts are that many people who begin to drink continue to do so until they are either drunk or develop a high tolerance for alcohol intake. According to the U.S. government's National Institute on Alcohol Abuse and Alcoholism roughly 1 in 7 of the nation's 100 million drinkers has alcohol-related health problems. Knowing these facts should alert us to the potential deleterious effects of this substance. Certainly, wine should be avoided whenever consumption would put the individual or others at risk. This includes times of pregnancy and when driving.

Wine, like herbs, must be used with knowledge and with caution. It is not a substance to be abused, but one to use with conscious choice and for purposes of relaxation or medicinal applications.

WINE AS A FOOD

Wine is an alcoholic beverage made from fermented grape juice. Wines are colored red, white, or rose and are labeled as dry, medium, or sweet. They fall into three basic categories: natural or "table" wines, which have an alcohol content of 8 to 14 percent; sparkling wines, such as champagne, which have an alcohol content similar to table wines and which contain carbon dioxide; and fortified wines, which have an alcohol content of 15 to 24 percent, and are drunk either as aperitifs or with dessert, depending on their sweetness. The various types of fortified wines include sherry, port, and aromatic wines and bitters such as vermouth.

Traditionally, we serve wine at the table where it is used as a food along with other foods. Because of the presence of organic acids, tannins, and other components, our bodies absorb the alcohol in wine much more slowly than the alcohol in other alcoholic solutions. We usually sip wine with our meals, resulting in still slower absorption of the alcohol, yielding relatively low and safe blood-alcohol concentrations.

Red wine should be served at room temperature, while white and rosé wines should be chilled prior to drinking. An

Oriental version of wine, sake (sah'-kee), is a sweet and color-less fermented wine. Often called Japanese rice wine, it has a high alcoholic content (12 to 16 percent by volume) and none of the carbon dioxide found in other fermented drinks such as beer. Sake is made from rice that is cleaned, steamed, treated with a special yeast, and allowed to ferment for 4 to 5 weeks. Near the end of the fermentation, more rice and water are added, and a second fermentation takes place. The resulting liquor is drawn off, filtered, and placed in casks for maturing. It is served warm in a small table container, poured into thimble-size cups and sipped. Table 16.1 details the calorie content of major wine types, while table 16.2 details some wine food facts.

WINE	Cal/100 cc.	Cal/oz.	Serving (oz.)	Cal/typical serving
Red Table Wines				
Burgundy	80.2	24.1	4	96.4
Cabernet	82.8	24.8	4	99.2
Chianti	81.8	24.5	4	98.0
Claret	79.8	23.9	4	95.6
Zinfandel	81.8	23.5	4	94.0
Rosé Table Wines	78.3	23.5	4	94.0
White Table Wines				
Chablis	73.8	22.1	4	88.4
Champagne	82.5	24.8	4	99.2
Rhine	76.7	23.0	4	92.0
Riesling	74.8	22.4	4	89.6
Dry sauterne	74.8	23.2	4	89.6
Sauterne	77.2	23.2	4	92.8
Sweet sauterne	87.1	26.1	4	104.4
Cocktail and Dessert Wines				
Red port	161.3	48.4	2	96.8
White port	150.0	45.0	2	90.0
Muscatel	163.2	49.0	2	98.0
Dry sherry	130.1	39.0	2	78.0
Sweet sherry	152.7	45.8	2	91.6
Dry vermouth	113.2	34.0	2	102.0
Sweet vermouth	150.4	45.1	2	135.3

▬▬▬

TABLE 16.1   *Calorie Content of Major Wine Types*

1. Wine is technically a food, a source of energy for work and body maintenance.

2. In moderate quantities, wine has no deleterious effect on growth or development, but it is not recommended during pregnancy.

3. The content of B vitamins and minerals in wine make it a desirable supplemental source of these substances in daily diets.

4. Most wines may be effectively incorporated into low-sodium diets.

5. Wine resembles gastric juice more closely than does any other natural beverage.

6. In moderate amounts, wine stimulates gastric secretion and motility, increases bile flow, and assists the natural processes of evacuation of the colon.

TABLE 16.2   Wine Food Facts

WINE AS AN ENERGY SOURCE

Wine supplies useful energy, mostly from alcohol at the rate of approximately 7 calories per gram and from carbohydrates at the rate of 4 calories per gram. Table wines average about 80 calories per 100 cc. or 24 calories per oz., while cocktail and dessert wines average about 150 calories per 100 cc. or 45 calories per oz.

CASE STUDY | *Agnes*

Agnes was 32 years old. She had been divorced for two years and was conspicuously underweight. It seemed no matter how she tried, Agnes could not muster the desire to eat. Six months ago, she quit her job and went back home to Mississippi to live with her parents. They tried to help her shake her depression and helped care for her ten-year-old son. They made every attempt to entice their daughter to eat their pancake and bacon breakfasts and old-fashioned meat and potato dinners. Despite their best efforts, Agnes had no appetite. She simply would not eat. All she did was mope around the house sipping glass after glass of iced tea and feeling sorry for herself.

Two weeks after Agnes had moved back with her parents, a neighbor invited her to visit. During the visit, she was offered a glass of sherry. She accepted it and found that the salutary effects caused her to stay longer than she had intended. She even indulged in a plate of sandwiches that her hostess offered during their enjoyable visit. They had so much fun that Agnes agreed to return to pick up where they left off.

When she returned, she once again accepted a glass of sherry. To her surprise, not only did she eat the plate of sandwiches but also accepted and enjoyed a piece of carrot cake. She returned home happy, satisfied, and full. In fact, she got along with the neighbor so well that they decided to make a biweekly routine of their afternoon rendezvous. The next week Agnes discovered that the Tuesday and Friday visits were the highlight of her week. She felt like she had met someone with whom she had something in common, and after each visit, she returned home feeling relaxed and full.

Within two weeks, she began to make a correlation between the sherry and her appetite, so she decided to try the experiment at home with her dad. Sure enough, it seemed to make a difference. She soon accepted the fact that with a glass of sherry before meals, she relaxed more, stopped thinking about her miserable situation, and actually had an appetite for dinner. At the same time, she decided to follow her mother's advice and stop drinking the iced tea all afternoon. Within a month's time, her anorexia abated and she began putting on some much needed weight.

Observation

In people suffering from anorexia and/or loss of weight, wine intake has a double beneficial effect: calorie intake and relaxation. Goetzl (1953) reported on a series of patients whose average caloric intake was increased by 60 percent over a three-month period, accompanied by a 12 percent increase in body weight. Wine stimulates the appetite directly through its physiological effect on the buccal mucosa. Based on laboratory studies, the wine components of acetic, tartaric, and tannic acids have been reported to have a specific appetite-stimulating action (Irvin, Ahokas, & Goetzl, 1950). In general, relatively small amounts of wine preceding and during mealtimes stimulate the appetite by physiological as well as psychological means (Dufour, Archer, & Gordis, 1992). However, ingestion of larger quantities, especially during a prolonged period before meals, may depress the appetite and promote drinking rather than eating. Appetite stimulation and relaxation are, of course, the goal for people like Agnes.

USE IN WEIGHT REDUCTION

Wine can also play a role in the control of obesity, especially when emotional tension is a contributory factor in the overeating. For many of us, a reducing diet is easy to come by, easy to understand, but extremely difficult to follow. Lolli's studies have shown that the appropriate use of wine can contribute to a weight reduction program by making it easier for us to adhere to a prescribed diet. Amounts proposed for this purpose range from 6 to 8 ounces of dry wine, taken approximately half an hour before the major meal of the day. Use before bedtime may reduce insomnia, lessening the craving for a bedtime snack (Balboni, 1963). When a dry wine was incorporated into a reducing diet, investigators demonstrated that most subjects naturally decreased their carbohydrate intake (Lolli, 1963).

MEDICINAL USE IN ILLNESS AND DISEASE

It is interesting to note that there is scant reference regarding the medicinal use of wine from 1960 to 1990. Reference to wine or alcohol in the journals during the past three decades has focused on alcohol addiction and its treatment. Hence, many of us have not been exposed to the beneficial effects of this food. Only since 1990 have we begun to see a resurgence in published reports regarding the benefits of wine.

Emotional Tension

The most obvious site of action of wine is in the central nervous system. We need not be skilled in psychology to note the effects of moderate quantities of wine at social gatherings. The speech and bearing of people and the play of features bear witness to its power. Restraints are removed, overly acute sensibilities are blunted, and little excitabilities are smoothed. Ideas and mental images follow each other with greater rapidity. A "cerebral sense of richness" occurs and lastly, a condition of euphoria and a more serene state of consciousness ensues. This statement, which may have been made by any observer today was, in fact, made more than 90 years ago (Billings, 1903). In slightly different forms, it has been made by others 600 years ago and even several millennia ago (Lucia, 1963).

Coronary Heart Disease

The heart is a primary focal area for the medicinal use of wine. Relief from anginal pain with wine, cordials, and brandy has been regularly reported since the observations of Heberden (1786) in the eighteenth century. When health care providers worked with angina patients during the 1950s, alcoholic beverages ranked second only to nitrates in controling this symptom (White, 1951). I remember well working evenings on the medical wards in a large hospital in New York City during the late 1960s and passing out many 2-ounce cups of brandy or sherry to our cardiac patients. We routinely kept the bottles in the medicine cabinet with the other generic medications. Remember, those were the days before unit dose and pharmacy preparation of medications. Looking at this from within the framework of a lifetime, it was not so long ago. But the fact of the matter is, it worked. It was inexpensive and easy to dispense. Patients not only got the vasodilation effect but also seemed to relax and sleep better.

Current literature is less romantic and more factual. The relationship between alcohol consumption and angiographically documented coronary artery disease was examined among 484 men who underwent coronary arteriography. A decrease in the average coronary artery disease scores was observed with increasing alcohol consumption until a mean consumption of about 100 ml. per day. These findings provide additional evidence that the reduction of the clinical coronary risk observed in moderate alcohol consumers might be secondary, at least partly, to an anatomically less extensive disease (Ducimetiere et al., 1993).

Other recent studies have put forth the hypothesis that the presence of trans-reveratrol in red wine may be related to some of its therapeutic properties (Mattivi, 1993). The "French paradox" (apparent compatibility of a high-fat diet with a low incidence of coronary atherosclerosis) has been attributed to the regular drinking of red wine. However, the alcohol content of wine may not be the sole explanation for this protection. Red wine contains phenolic compounds, and the antioxidant properties of these may have an important role. In in-vitro studies with phenolic substances in red wine and normal human low-density lipoprotein (LDL), researchers found that red wine inhibits the copper-catalyses oxidation of LDL. Wine diluted 1,000-fold and containing 10 millimoles/L total phenolics inhibited LDL oxidation significantly more than alpha-tocopherol. The findings show that the nonalcoholic components of red wine have potent antioxidant properties toward oxidation of human LDL (Frankel et al., 1993; "Inhibition of LDL," 1993).

Epidemiological studies indicate that the consumption of alcohol at the level of intake in France (20 to 30 grams per day or two to three 4-ounce servings per day) can reduce the risk of coronary heart disease (CHD) by at least 40 percent. Alcohol is believed to protect from CHD by preventing atherosclerosis through the action of high-density-lipoprotein cholesterol, but serum concentrations of this factor are no higher in France than in other countries. Re-examination of previous results suggests that moderate alcohol intake does not prevent CHD through an effect on atherosclerosis, but rather through a hemostatic mechanism. Data from Wales show that platelet aggregation, which is related to CHD, is inhibited significantly by alcohol at levels of intake associated with reduced risk of CHD. Inhibition of platelet reactivity by wine may be one explanation for protection from CHD in France, since pilot studies have shown that platelet reactivity is lower in France than in Scotland (Renaud, 1992).

Other Conditions

During our lifetime, wine has been found to be beneficial in a host of other conditions. These include renal disease, infectious diseases, Parkinsonism, gout, and viral hepatitis. However, even though we know that wine does have beneficial effects, some cautions are advisable. First, we all know the potentially deadly effects of overconsumption and addiction. All kinds of alcohol addiction programs and support groups have arisen over the past three decades to combat alcohol abuse. The caution with wine, as with most other areas of life, is to use it in moderation. Too much can be detrimental.

Cautions:

The second caution relates to women. Recent studies report a positive correlation between alcohol consumption and breast cancer. A United States Nurses' Health Study in 1986 examined alcohol consumption in relation to risk of breast cancer via dietary questionnaires that were administered both before and after diagnosis. Analysis of the data demonstrated an elevated risk of breast cancer among women who drank 30 grams or more of alcohol daily (about two drinks) as compared to nondrinkers (Giovannucci et al., 1993). In another questionnaire study done in Spain, data suggested that even at moderate levels of alcohol intake (less than 8 grams per day), a 50 percent increase in risk of breast cancer was found. Consumption of 20 grams or more of alcohol per day was associated with a 70-percent elevation in breast cancer risk compared with that of nondrinkers (Martin-Moreno, 1993). The significant thing to note in both of these studies, however, is that no differentiation was made regarding the kind of alcohol consumed. Alcohols in beverages such as bourbon, scotch, and rum are of a different substance and potency than the alcohol in wines.

The differences among the types of alcohol become apparent upon analysis. In a study of age-specific consumption of beer, wine, and liquor and the occurrence of disease, the findings were noteworthy. Overall, there was a modest indication that high levels of alcohol consumption (11 or more drinks per week) were associated with increased risk of large bowel cancer. In site-specific analyses, only rectal cancer demonstrated a significant linear trend with increasing consumption. Beer was associated significantly with rectal cancer. Wine consumption was associated inversely with rectal cancers. These relationships appeared to be consistent for recent, past, and total lifetime consumption and were not attributable to differences in dietary habits (Newcomb, Storer, & Marcus, 1993). Again, care must be taken to differentiate between not only the amount, but the type of alcohol consumed.

SUMMARY

Table wines have been with us since time immemorial. Wine is a food that when consumed in moderation can be beneficial as a relaxant or as a stimulant, depending upon the setting and the type of wine ingested. Some people like to think of wine as a fruited beverage because it is in fact derived from grapes. Wine may be used as a healing food when taken with a sense of consciousness and care.

References

Balboni, C. (1963). Alcohol in relation to dietary patterns. In S. P. Lucia (Ed.), *Alcohol and civilization.* New York: McGraw-Hill.

Billings, J. S., et al. (1903). *Physiological aspects of liquor problems.* New York: Houghton Mifflin.

Ducimetiere, P., Guize, L., Marciniak, A., Milton, H., Richard, J., & Rufat, P. (1993). Arteriographically documented coronary artery disease and alcohol consumption in French men. *European Heart Journal, 14* (6), 727–733.

Dufour M. C., Archer L., & Gordis, E. (1992). Alcohol and the elderly. *Clinical Geriatric Medicine, 8* (1), 127–141.

Frankel, E. N., Kanner, J., German, J. B., Parks, E., & Kinsella, J. E. (1993). Inhibition of oxidation of human low-density lipoprotein by phenolic substances in red wine. *Lancet, 341,* 454–457.

Giovannucci, E., et al. (1993). Recall and selection bias in reporting past alcohol consumption. *Cancer Causes Control, 4* (5), 441–448.

Goetzl, F. R. (1953). *A note on the possible usefulness of wine in the management of anorexia.* Oakland, CA: Permanente Foundation.

Heberden, W. (1786). Some account of a disorder of the breast. *Medical Transcriptions of the Royal College of Physicians in London, 2,* 59–67.

Inhibition of LDL oxidation by phenolic substances in red wine: A clue to the French paradox? (1993). *Nutrition Review, 51* (6), 185–187.

Irvin, D. L., Ahokas, A. J., & Goetzl, F. R. (1950). The influence of ethyl alcohol in low concentrations upon olfactory acuity and the sensation complex of appetite and satiety. *Permanente Foundation Medical Bulletin, 8,* 97–101.

Lolli, G. (1963). The role of wine in the treatment of obesity. *New York State Journal of Medicine, 62,* 3438–3443.

Lolli, G., Serianni, E., Golder, G., Mariani, A., & Toner, M. (1952). Relationships between intake of carbohydrate-rich foods and intake of wine and other alcoholic beverages. *Quarterly Journal Studies Alcohol, 13,* 401–420.

Lucia, S. P. (1963). The Antiquity of Alcohol in Diet and Medicine. In S.P. Lucia (Ed.), *Alcohol and civilization.* New York: McGraw-Hill.

Martin-Moreno, J., et al. (1993). Alcoholic beverage consumption and risk of breast cancer in Spain. *Cancer Causes Control, 4* (4), 345–353.

Mattivi, F. (1993). Solid phase extraction of trans-reveratrol from wines for HPLC analysis. *Z Lebensm Unter Forsch, 196* (6), 522–525.

Newcomb, P., Storer, B., & Marcus, P. (1993). Cancer of the large bowel in women in relation to alcohol consumption: A case control study in Wisconsin. *Cancer Causes Control, 4* (5), 405–411.

Renaud, S. (1992). Wine, alcohol, platelets, and the French paradox for coronary heart disease. *Lancet, 339,* 1523–1526.

White, P. D. (1951). *Heart disease.* New York: Macmillan.

17 CONTROVERSIES IN NUTRITION

Each of the following areas of nutrition can be classified as controversial. Despite the widespread approval of these issues by some caregivers, others continue to be skeptical.

MEGAVITAMIN THERAPY

Megavitamin therapy is the name of a controversial mode of nutrient therapy that involves the ingestion of large doses of vitamins. Linus Pauling was the first to use the term *orthomolecular* to characterize the treatment of human disease with nutrients that naturally occur in the human body. The basic premise of orthomolecular medicine is that the greatest long-term health benefits in disease treatment are derived from establishing the concentration of essential nutrients in the body. This is done by adjusting diets, eliminating junk foods, and, most controversially, ingesting large (mega) doses of various nutrients. Pauling became best known when he advocated large intakes (megadoses) of vitamin C for treatment of the common cold.

Orthomolecular medicine is primarily utilized in the treatment of psychiatric disorders. Initially used to treat schizophrenia, the scope of disorders thought to improve with the application of orthomolecular principles has continually broadened. It includes, for example, epilepsy, autism, senility, arthritis, and allergies. Orthomolecular therapy is also used to treat diseases and chronic problems such as backaches and psoriasis.

While treatment programs vary, the main focus is on megavitamin therapy followed by a combination of other essential nutrients that are lacking or inadequate in the body. Drugs are used infrequently, the goal being to subsist on nutrients alone. Treatment programs are developed through clinical tests, psychiatric examinations, and consultation to identify the different nutrient requirements of each patient. Some believe, although this is highly controversial, that awareness of drug side effects and the desire for natural treatments will make orthomolecular medicine a dominant therapeutic tool of the future.

FOOD ADDITIVES

A food additive is a nonfood substance added to food during processing to preserve or improve its color, texture, flavor, or value. By definition, the class also includes substances that may indirectly become components of food. For example, a chemical used to make cereal packaging paper is considered a food additive if the packaged cereal absorbs even minute quantities of the additive.

Iron, minerals, and vitamins are regularly introduced into foods to compensate for losses during processing or to provide additional nutrients. Iodine may be added to salt, vitamin A to margarine, and vitamin D to milk. Flavoring agents, including salts, spices, essential oils, and natural and synthetic flavors, make up the largest single class of additives. Additives that improve texture include emulsifiers, stabilizers, and thickeners. Gums, dextrins, and starches are used to give more substance to soups and desserts. Pectin and gelatin are added to thicken jams and jellies. Lecithin is the primary emulsifier used in salad dressings and chocolates.

The additives used to preserve food are primarily chemical antimicrobial agents such as the benzoates, propionates, and sorbates that retard spoilage caused by bacteria, yeasts, and molds.

Antioxidants are used to keep fats and oils from spoiling and to prevent discoloration of smoked or canned meats. Ascorbic acid is used to prevent the discoloration of canned fruits.

The wide use of synthetic additives is a twentieth-century phenomenon associated with the growth of the food industry. Some of the additives used today are labeled in the terminology of the Food and Drug Administration (FDA) as "Generally Recognized As Safe" (GRAS). A number of these substances had been used before 1958 when amendments to the Food, Drug, and Cosmetic Act required that new food additives be tested for safety with no recorded evidence of harmful effects. Others were given GRAS status after 1958. Synthetic food colors have also come under FDA scrutiny, and some dyes are now prohibited as food additives. In 1986, the FDA banned sulfites for use as color preservatives in fresh fruits and vegetables. The FDA had previously required labeling of sulfite contents in other foods.

Concern is also growing about chemicals that indirectly find their way into foods by way of pesticide residues on fruits and vegetables or through medications and stimulants given to animals. In 1979, the FDA banned the use of the synthetic hormone diethylstilbestrol in cattle because residues were showing up in meat products. In the early 1990s, the FDA and other federal agencies responsible for food safety increased the amount of testing being performed for pesticides.

ORGANICALLY GROWN FOODS

Organically grown foods are foods that are grown without the use of chemical fertilizers or pesticides. Natural foods are usually thought of as foods processed without chemical additives.

Interest in organically grown foods has developed rapidly in the United States since studies in the 1960s linked certain food additives with cancer and other diseases. It is widely acknowledged that some pesticides used on crops and some chemicals used in food processing may be harmful to our health. However, for many chemicals, health hazards have not been proved, nor has it been proved that organically grown foods are nutritionally superior to those grown using chemical fertilizers.

FOOD IRRADIATION

After 40 years of experimentation and controversy over the nutritional and environmental safety implications of preserving and disinfecting foods with radioactive materials, food irradiation has become a reality. Essentially, food irradiation is a process in which food is exposed to gamma radiation from radioactive materials such as cobalt 60 or cesium-137 or through linear accelerator electron beams to kill bacteria, insects, or parasites that may be present.

Although the doses used on food are too weak to actually make the food radioactive, they are strong enough to disrupt the chemical bonds that hold molecules together, thus killing or inhibiting the growth of organisms that cause disease, spoilage, and other forms of deterioration. A typical chest x-ray delivers a dose of 1/100 of 1 rad (radiation absorbed dose). In contrast, the amount of energy used in food irradiation, measured in units called "Grays," is considerably higher—100,000 rads = 1,000 Grays = 1 kiloGray (1kGy). One kiloGray increases the shelf life of some fruits and vegetables by changing the chemistry of their cells to retard ripening and rotting. Higher doses, 4.75 to 8 kiloGrays, kill salmonella. Very high doses, up to the 30 kGy used to irradiate herbs and spices, render foods sterile.

Food irradiation in the United States was developed primarily at government expense. It started with post-World War II research by the United States army to create good-tasting, economical, shelf-stable field rations for the troops. Interest in food irradiation research and development further expanded in both the government and private sectors during the early to mid 1950s.

Progress slowed somewhat after the passage of the Food Additives Amendment to the Federal Food, Drugs, and Cosmetic Act in 1958. In the amendment, Congress and administrative agencies classified irradiation as a food additive rather than a process since its use affects the characteristics of foods. Therefore, companies wishing to use irradiation were required to petition the FDA for approval. The new use of radiation had to be proven safe with appropriate toxicological studies.

The first approved uses of irradiation occurred in 1963 to preserve canned bacon and to kill insects in wheat and wheat products. In 1964, irradiation of potatoes was allowed to retard sprouting. However, bacon regulations were revoked in 1968 when further evaluation of the data raised doubts that the safety of radiation-sterilized bacon had been demonstrated.

The FDA established the Bureau of Foods Irradiated Food Committee in 1979 to review the agency's policies regarding irradiation and to recommend how to test more accurately for the effects of food irradiation. The committee estimated that a 1 kGy irradiation dose would form "radiolytic products," a class of molecules formed when the ions produced by radiation react with other molecules in the food. Ten percent of these molecules would be unknown compounds. Despite the fact that it takes only one mutant molecule to start a cancer, the committee concluded that at doses below 1kGy, any single "unique" radiolytic product of unusual toxicity would be negligible.

Because it is impossible to test food for the amount of radiation administered, the committee conceded to base their evaluation of irradiation primarily on theoretical estimates extrapolated from radiation chemistry. In 1981, the FDA completely reversed its testing policy, concluding that an adequate margin of safety had been demonstrated for foods irradiated below 1 kGy. Consequently, without the burden of testing, new uses of food irradiation are approved more quickly. To date, approval has been given to irradiate pork, fresh fruits and vegetables, dry or dehydrated enzyme preparations, herbs and spices, and most recently, poultry.

ARTIFICIAL SWEETENERS

Artificial sweeteners such as saccharin, cyclamates, and aspartame were developed to replace naturally occurring sugars in food products. In 1981, the FDA banned cyclamates and enforced controls on the use of saccharin. It approved the sale of aspartame, a product 200 times as sweet as sucrose.

Aspartame is formed by joining two amino acids that are naturally produced by the bacterial breakdown of organic substances. Aspartame has a brief and controversial past. It was accidentally discovered in 1965 when the substance was being studied as a potential ulcer treatment. The U.S. FDA rescinded its original 1974 approval following controversial reports that aspartame, when used to combat obesity, caused brain lesions in laboratory animals. In light of controversies over other artificial sweeteners, chiefly cyclamates and saccharin, the FDA conducted several more years of extensive tests. Aspartame was granted limited approval in 1981 and final approval in 1983. It quickly became an ingredient in many diet foods, especially soft drinks. It is now one of the most frequently used sweeteners in the marketplace.

As you can see, any of these artificial sweeteners can cause problems. However, it is theorized that more people in the United States currently die of obesity-related diseases than of ones related to artificial sweeteners. It is best to limit both your sugar and artificial sweetener consumption, not to choose one over the other.

SUMMARY

Controversy abounds in a world of change. It is a part of the nature of change. When controversy stirs, remember that most fruitful discoveries that have advanced our civilization have occurred in the midst of controversy. However, despite the seal of approval bestowed on controversial products or issues, it is probably best to use these and other artificial substances in moderate to small amounts.

GAINING
CONTROL OF
YOUR WEIGHT

18 EFFECTIVE DIETING

Do diets really work? This may be the most perplexing question of the decade. There are literally hundreds of diet plans and countless thousands of people who are on "diets" at this very moment. The unfortunate fact is that 95 percent of them will regain all their lost weight, with proportionately more fat than muscle.

What keeps dieters ready and willing to spend their time, money, and energy on yet another diet is the addictive short-term, rapid weight loss that is possible with virtually every diet in the marketplace. For an idea of the breadth and range of popular diet books, go to any bookstore and look at the titles. At one store I visited recently, there must have been 30 titles devoted to diets alone.

HOW FAD DIETS WORK

During the first few days of a severely reduced-calorie diet, weight seemingly drops off at a substantially satisfying rate. But instead of losing fat, our bodies are consuming their temporary energy reserve (glycogen), which weighs about a pound, and when associated water, weighs another 3 to 4 pounds. The temporary diet is over when our hunger returns and the glycogen is restored as soon as we consume food. Our bodies then readjust for the water deficit, and we regain the weight just as quickly as it was lost.

Any diet that promises a weight loss of more than 1 to 2 pounds per week is either counting on this very temporary rapid weight loss or on a prolonged diet plan that restricts calories below 1,200, the minimum amount we need for basic metabolic processes. While it is possible to increase metabolism to help whittle away stored fat calories, severely restricting intake is not the way to do it.

One of the primary determinants of the body's basal metabolic rate is the proportion of lean muscle to fat tissue. Each pound of muscle burns 30 to 50 calories a day to stay alive, while fat burns only 2 calories per pound a day. When a diet offers too few calories to support basal metabolic rate, our bodies choose to hold on to precious fat molecules for what they perceive to be famine times ahead and switch to lean muscle tissue for fuel. Consequently, our metabolic rate slackens to conserve energy for this new survival mode. Restricted food intake also supplies inadequate nutrients for optimum health and energy.

POPULAR DIET PLANS

It is not within the scope or intent of this book to elaborate on specific diets, but it is important to realize that thousands, perhaps millions of people, currently follow one or more of the well-known diet plans. You probably have heard of some of them or maybe even tried one or more of them yourself. Pritikin, Weight Watchers, Jenny Craig, and the grapefruit diet plan are examples of but a few. Some of these popular commercial diet programs do work toward whole body health by advocating exercise and/or stress management programs along with their eating plan. Some of the more intriguing programs and their lively leaders, such as Susan Powter, advocate complete lifestyle change to remake ourselves. The point to remember here is that some of these diets do work for some people. Not all of us are alike, however, so many of us need to look in alternative directions.

Some people find that the Dean Ornish diet for a healthy heart works for them. Basically a macrobiotic (meatless) diet,

Ornish teaches converts to eliminate meat fat and most sugars while incorporating an exercise and stress management plan. Other nutritionists such as Jeffrey Bland and Jonathan Wright have developed their own specialty diet regimens. Each of these plans works for some people, especially the ones who are serious about weight management.

PERMANENT WEIGHT LOSS

If you are serious about permanent weight loss and weight maintenance, you do not want a quick-fix, weight reduction plan. Instead you must employ all your body-mind-spirit resources to change or modify your lifestyle. Weight loss without long-term behavior change will fail. The weight will return and the roller coaster process will begin anew. A diet plan that includes exercise, a change in attitudes, and an alteration in causative behaviors is the only thing that will work for the long term. Implementing a plan of healing nutrition into a healthy life plan can bring about miraculous whole body changes.

BREAKING OLD HABITS, SUBSTITUTING NEW BEHAVIORS

Behavioral therapists say that it takes 21 days to develop a new habit. Just as it is easier to sew an entirely new dress than remake an old one, it takes longer to tear apart old ingrained, bad habits and rebuild them than it does to begin from scratch. So it is with our eating habits. If, for example, you have been drinking caffeinated soft drinks, eating donuts for mid-morning snacks, and having your main meal in the evening for a decade or more, it may take a while to change this routine.

Willpower

Willpower is one of the most important aspects of dieting. Willpower is what makes diets work and what helps us to achieve what we want. Let us talk about willpower and food and willpower and emotions. What does the word *willpower* really mean? Does it mean that we have to deny ourselves time to relax at the end of the day because we have to jog to keep our bodies exercised to live longer? Does it mean we cannot go to an afterhours party because we promised to take the kids to a ball game? Or does it simply mean determination?

I propose that willpower is what we use to get ahead in life. Willpower is what we use along with determination, whether it be to get our bodies healthy or to make a million dollars. We all know people who constantly complain about their weight, their diets, or their lives. Those of us who have willpower do something about the situation. For example, we might throw out the junk food in our cabinets or go skating or dancing if we are dieting. Willpower is what will change our lives and our eating habits. We have all heard this before, yet it is a true statement. We must have willpower to succeed.

How do we get willpower to diet? First, let's talk of situations. You are sitting at the table tonight and you have made or bought a cake for dessert. Go ahead, have a small piece. When you want another, just say this word loud and clear in your head—*no*! Put the dessert in the freezer or give it away. Go on with life, and within a day you will have forgotten it. At this point, start saying no to other high-fat, high-calorie foods. By doing this, you will begin saying yes to a lot more.

This is the only life you have, unless you believe in reincarnation, and of course, you want to make the best of it. By making yourself what you want to be, you will know and be satisfied that you have accomplished something. Although it may seem strange to find a willpower chapter in a book on nutrition, this book is not just about food, it is about you. You must look at every aspect of yourself to understand the relationship between food and yourself and how to develop the willpower to control it. Try the following steps to boost your willpower:

1. Think about what you really want.

2. Think about why you want it.

3. Realize that willpower is your way to get it, whether it is a lower weight or a healthier body.

4. Do what you know is best, not what your taste buds tell you.

Creative Visualization

A creative way to follow through on willpower is to utilize an imagery or visualization experience before you eat. Try this exercise prior to your next meal.

Take a long, slow, deep breath in through your nose. Hold your breath as you count to four, and then exhale through your mouth. As you follow this breathing pattern one more time, read the following script:

- I am totally and completely relaxed.

- I am losing from 2 to 7 pounds per month. I am losing weight consistently until I reach my goal.

- I am eating less and enjoying it more.

- Both my appetite and hunger are satisfied quickly.

- I am leaving food on my plate and feel good about it.

- I am losing pounds consistently each month until I reach my weight goal.

- I can see myself as I will look when I reach my ideal weight.

- All these suggestions are becoming a part of me and are effective now.

Food Diary

It is often difficult to recall just what you ate and when you ate it. Attempting to recall specific foods at specific times may block your ability to relate eating behaviors to being overweight. Before beginning to diet, as well as once you are underway, you will probably find it helpful to record what you eat. In this way, you will have an hour-by-hour record of what you actually ate, not just what you remember. It is amazing how easily we can forget the actual quantities and types of food we ate just 24 hours ago. A food diary recording is an excellent guide for you as you begin to modify eating behaviors. Table 18.1 depicts a simple recording schedule that you can copy into a notebook. The idea is simply to put in writing everything that you put into your mouth. This is the only way you can really know your actual intake.

Date	Time	Food Consumed
	6:00	
	7:00	
	8:00	
	9:00	
	10:00	
	11:00	
	Noon	
	1:00	
	2:00	
	3:00	
	4:00	
	5:00	
	6:00	
	7:00	
	8:00	
	9:00	
	10:00	
	11:00	
	Midnight	
	12:00 A.M.–6:00 A.M.	

TABLE 18.1   Food Diary

Food Cravings

Sometimes despite our best intentions, it seems impossible to apply willpower when we crave high-calorie foods.

CASE STUDY | *Betty*

Betty worked nights in the hospital telemetry unit. She had been out of school for three years and, much to her chagrin, had gained 60 pounds. When she met with the wellness nurse for the first time, she did not intend to delve into her nutritional habits. She simply wanted a quick physical assessment and the okay to begin an exercise class. The wellness nurse strongly suggested that in addition to the exercise class, Betty return for weekly nutritional counseling sessions.

During the weekly sessions, Betty's eating patterns unfolded. After work at 7:00 A.M., she went home, made breakfast for her family, and got the children off to school. Then she ate the leftovers, cleaned the kitchen, and went to bed. She was up at 4:00 P.M. to greet the kids with an afternoon snack. Later, she made supper and ate a leisurely meal with her family. The nurse counselor soon discovered that the problem eating time came during the night. By the time Betty arrived at work, she had met all her caloric requirements for the day. Betty and her nurse colleagues had started working the same shift at the same time and had worked together continuously for three years. They had acquired the pattern of each one bringing in a covered dish every night so they could eat a communal "supper" at 2:00 A.M. and pastries before the last flurry of activities at 5:00 A.M. They also drank copious quantities of coffee throughout the night. To add spice to their lives, they "dressed up" their coffee with fancy commercial creams. They took turns bringing in the cream. As you might suspect, the dairy creamers got fancier and fancier. At first they used nondairy creamer, then half and half, but a year ago they began using the speciality coffee creamers in the pint-size milk cartons. Amaretto, Irish Cream, and Swiss Mocha flavors were among their favorites. The craving for coffee and creamers became an unconscious addiction. Without thinking, Betty added the creamers to her coffee at home and insisted on real cream in her coffee when she ate out.

It was not until the nurse counselor explained the high-fat, high-calorie content to Betty that she became aware of how much additional intake she was consuming. Betty reported her insights to her colleagues on the unit and solicited their input for dieting strategies. They too had become fat.

The group devised a plan for cream elimination and gradual coffee withdrawal. Since they realized they had all developed both caffeine and fat addictions, they agreed to tackle the problem together. Over a three-month period, they substituted skim milk for cream, changed to low-calorie nutritional snacks to replace their 2:00 A.M. "supper," and replaced their caffeinated coffee with decaffeinated. After six months, they had completely revolutionized their nighttime eating habits and had begun to shed pounds. Two of the three nurses also began exercise classes to augment the new lifestyle.

Observation

Cravings usually creep up on us. Our insidious behaviors can develop into food addictions without our realizing what is happening. The following list of activities may help to combat food cravings:

1. Bring the food craving into conscious awareness.
2. Begin a food diary to decipher what events trigger the eating behavior.
3. Try to sublimate the desire to eat into another productive behavior. When the desire to eat a high-fat food strikes you, be prepared in advance to substitute another activity or desire. For example, if you have been wanting to take a weekend trip but cannot afford it, start saving money. Each time you want to spend 50 cents on a candy bar or soft drink, put

the money in your portable piggy bank instead. You may be surprised at how quickly the funds add up and how soon you will be able to reward yourself because of the substituted behavior.

4. Volunteer to work in a soup kitchen or homeless shelter. Spend a shift or two a week serving meals to the down and out. The psychological impact of this technique has proved beneficial for many who are breaking food craving patterns.

WHEN AND HOW TO DIET

There are numerous ways to diet. The one you choose will depend on your personality type. In this section, we will see how dieting worked for several different people.

Dieting Alone

A way that works well for some is the isolation method. Those who follow this route virtually retreat from their everyday lives, buy a quantity of diet food, and do not go out.

CASE STUDY | Laura

Laura was an active head nurse on an oncology unit. In addition to her high-pressure job, she was the single parent of two teenage girls. Despite the nagging efforts of her slender daughters, Laura could not summon the willpower to stop eating. At work she was bombarded by the sweets left by well-meaning families and pastries served at staff parties and meetings. In the evenings at home, she was tired and felt she needed a good supper with her daughters. While trying to relax at night, she was exposed to television advertisements for foods and could not resist snacking and having an occasional mixed drink. After all, she was so tired and food was so comforting. Month after month, despite periodic attempts to diet, her overweight poundage persisted and some months she even gained weight.

One August, in a fury of disgust over what she had become, Laura made a rapid decision. She decided to get away from work, the kids, the house, and the TV and leave town. She recalled her misery following her divorce when the children were young. She remembered how her mother offered to keep the girls so that she could go on a vacation and snap out of her depression. It had worked. She had connected with a local scuba divers club organizing a group trip and had gone to a Mexican island to snorkle. She even had a miserable cold when she departed. The warm January sunshine, the tropical waters, and the group camaraderie had soon broken Laura's cold and the long-standing depression. She had been able to put her life problems into perspective, made new friends, and developed a new skill. By the end of the week, Laura had experienced a miraculous change in her body-mind-spirit health and returned to her home and career responsibilities with a new outlook.

Now, eight years later, Laura decided she needed another retreat from her immediate environment. This time she was not depressed, she was just fat. She asked one of her friends to look after the girls and arranged for leave from work. Since it was off-season, she was able to get good rates at a seaside resort close to the Mexican border in the same area where she had made a turn-around before. She loaded her car with a stock of good books, motivational tapes, and simple clothes. While driving to the beach, she crunched on carrot and celery sticks and rice cakes and drank one-calorie, caffeine-free, soft drinks.

Once in town, Laura ignored the billboards for fast foods and fancy seafood restaurants and drove directly to the grocery store. She stocked up on low-calorie drinks, fresh fruits and vegetables, fresh eggs, and low-calorie crunchy snacks. She bought no-fat, low-calorie margarine and breads to spread it on. She knew it would take a few days to shrink her massive stomach back to normal size, so she loaded up on foods that would contain bulk but not fats or calories. Armed with bags of diet groceries, Laura retreated to her seaside condominium and began her diet.

She figured that as long as she was retreating to diet she might as well work on her mental and spiritual health at the same time. She began to practice a meditation technique she had learned in college but never seemed to have time for in her busy life. In three days time, Laura read two novels, wrote three letters, swam in the pool, briskly walked the beach twice a day, and began to feel the lethargy ease from her heavy frame.

Television was declared a demon and she consciously unplugged it. She knew that the food ads broke even the most sterling willpower. She was determined not to succumb to the commercials designed to make America fat. She used her free evening time to stroll the beach and sit at the waves' edge to reflect on her past and contemplate her future.

On the fourth day, Laura awoke feeling invigorated. On this day, she developed a long-range planning schedule and then followed her previous days' routine.

On the fifth day, she tested herself in the outside world. She drove to a large public cafeteria for her major mid-day meal. Here she discovered she could buy any combination of four salads or vegetables for a modest price. Since she had declared this retreat week meatless, as well as alcoholfree, this was perfect. She purchased two salads, two hot vegetables, and a tall glass of un-iced water. Positioning herself at a window table, she ate slowly, savoring the hot vegetables. She ate the cold, crisp, carrot and raisin salad for dessert. She boxed the green salad to take home for the evening meal. Laura left the cafeteria full and happy. She had passed the test of the temptation to overindulge.

Laura rounded out the sixth day of her retreat beachcombing, swimming, and enjoying small portions of healthy, nutritious foods. On the seventh day, armed with carrots, celery, rice cakes, and a thermos of water, she drove back home. She felt psychologically stronger, mentally alert, spiritually attuned, and physically ready to begin a long-term eating program that would restore her to a state of vibrant health. She calculated that she spent $500 for the week and considered the cost well worth the self-esteem, self-confidence, and whole body health that she had generated.

Observation

Laura created a situation in which she could isolate herself from responsibilities in the fast-paced world and engage in a 7-day purification, renewal diet. She had the willpower to distance herself from alcohol, caffeine, and high-fat, high-calorie foods and the knowledge to choose what kinds of foods to eat. She created a support system by using motivational audio cassette tapes, withdrawing from television, and including the healing properties of a natural environment. Laura took no scale or measuring tape to monitor her progress because she knew she needed a long-term plan, not short-term calibrations.

For many, separation from the routine daily environment can make a significant difference. Thoughtful isolation can create the space to consider what got you into this condition in the first place and what forces you need in order to move to a more desirable state.

Dieting with a Buddy or Team

Most people are highly social beings and need the support of others to boost their willpower.

CASE STUDY | *Sandra*

Sandra was an evening staff nurse in the neonatal intensive care unit. She was in her thirties, unmarried, and was, by her own admission, in a rut. Two months ago she had broken off a long-term relationship with her live-in boyfriend. Neither he nor anything else in her life seemed to be on the right track. Since the breakup two months ago, Sandra had moped around with a sense of ennui and fatigue. Her overweight problem had not really concerned her until an event in the unit got her attention. Several overweight nurses from all the shifts in her unit decided to hold a contest. By the time the rules were established, ten nurses agreed to contribute $20 each and see who could lose the most weight in a three-month period. The winner would collect the $200 prize winnings. Sandra decided to join the pool. Perhaps she could finally concentrate and have a worthy personal goal.

All of the contestants weighed in and had their weight recorded every week. Several of the contestants teamed up together and developed a group strategy and plan. Sandra decided to go the Weight Watchers route. She went to their weekly meetings, bought their food, and became a true convert to their lifestyle change approach to the problem. They suggested she join a local exercise club. This caused her to change her daily schedule. Before she had slept from 2:00 A.M. to 10:00 A.M., had a leisurely breakfast, and watched TV before getting ready for work in the afternoon. After joining the exercise club, she changed her routine and began regular morning workout classes. She made new friends with other Weight Watcher associates and felt like she was starting her life all over again.

At the end of three months, Sandra won the contest. Not only had she lost the most weight in the group of her nursing colleagues, but she had established a network of new health-seeking friends. She collected the $200 prize and took her competitors out for an evening of miniature golf.

Observation

Sandra is typical of many of us. We eat and gain weight often without realizing how or when it happened. She was alert to the situation and seized the opportunity to do something about it. We all need social connections and friendships. We need to ensure that these social aspects enhance all areas of our lives.

EMPLOYING NEW STRATEGIES: COMPLEMENTARY HOLISTIC THERAPIES

When we decide to change our lifestyles and get serious about weight control we usually follow three routines:

1. We eat well-rounded, whole foods with minimal fat and sugar.

2. We begin a program of regular aerobic exercise and stretching.

3. We begin and follow a program of stress management.

Nurses with a holistic orientation will probably want to add some complementary therapies to this winning trio. Perhaps you will want to add guided imagery, touch, prayer and meditation, or music. These are but a few of the alternative therapies that, when used in conjunction with a program of healing nutrition, can empower our bodies, minds, and spirits.

SUMMARY

Dieting by itself is never a long-term answer to weight or health maintenance. To be effective, dieting must be accomplished by lifestyle changes that include exercise and stress management. When we become serious about weight loss, we must assess our entire being and, when we are truly ready, embark on a holistic lifestyle change program of whole-body healing.

I N D E X

A

Acid carbohydrates, 88
Acne, 24–25
Additives, food, 188–189
Adolescence, nutrition, 122–123
Adults, nutrition, 123
Algal polysaccharides, defined, 48
Allergies, 25
Aloe, 148
American Dietetic Association, vegetarianism and, 157
Amino acids, vegetarianism and, 158–159
Anemia, vegetarianism and, 155
Anger, 116
Aniseed, 148
Antioxidants, vitamins as, 99, 103
Artificial sweeteners, 191–192
Aspartame, 191
Attitudes, health and, 11–12

B

Backaches, orthomolecular medicine and, 188
Baking fish, 69
Balm, 149
Basil, 149
Bearberry, 149
Bioflavonoids, **102**
Biotin, **100**
Body-mind-spirit template, 4
Body odor, 25
Borage, 149
Breast cancer
   fats and, 84–85
   proteins and, 61
   wine and, 183–184

Broiling fish, 69
Bruises, 26
Bruxism, 26
Bureau of Foods Irradiated Food Committee, 191
Butter
   alternatives to, 83
   described, 82

C

Calcium, **106**
Calories
   content in common foods, **47**
   requirement for, 46
Cancer
   fats and, 84–85
   proteins and, 61
   wine and, 183–184
Capsules, described, 110
Caraway, 149
Carbohydrates
   addiction to, 94–95
   described, 87–88
Cardomon, 149
Cascara, 149
Cells, life of, 10–11
Cellular age, defined, 13
Cellulose, defined, 47
Chamomile, 149
Cheeses, 69–71
Chelated minerals, 104–105
Chemicals, composition of, 45–46
Chewable tablets, described, 110
Chloride, **106**
Cholesterol, 76–77